THE HORSE PHYSIOLOGY

Julie Brega

J.A. Allen
London

British Library Cataloguing in Publication Data
A catalogue record for this book is available
from the British Library

ISBN 0.85131.607.7

Published in Great Britain in 1995 by
J.A. Allen and Company Limited,
1 Lower Grosvenor Place,
Buckingham Palace Road,
London, SW1W 0EL.

Typeset in Hong Kong by Setrite Typesetters Ltd.
Printed in Hong Kong by Dah Hua Printing Press Co.

CONTENTS

LIST OF
ILLUSTRATIONS

ix

LIST OF
TABLES

ACKNOWLEDGEMENTS

I would like to thank the following friends for their invaluable help in the production of this book:

Debby Baker, for deciphering and typesetting the original manuscript.

Annalisa Barrelet, BVetMed, MS, Cert ESM, MRCVS, for veterinary editing and much expert advice.

Kitty Best, for the excellent illustrations.

Martin Diggle, for his patience and editing skills.

And special thanks to my family: to my parents, John and Sheila Hollywood, who look after our children, Holly and Josh, so brilliantly, allowing me to get some work done, to my step-daughter, Zoe, for keeping the horses, office and myself organized, and finally to my husband, Bill, for his constant help and support.

INTRODUCTION

The Horse: Physiology is one of six books in the Progressive Series. This series forms the basis of an advanced open learning course offered by The Open College of Equestrian Studies.

The main objective of these books is to present the information needed by the equestrian enthusiast in a clear and logical manner. This information is invaluable to everyone interested in horses, whether in a professional capacity as a yard manager or examination trainee, or as a private horse owner.

This book deals with the vast and fascinating subject of equine physiology — the way in which the horse's body works.

Starting with the formation and composition of bone, the skeletal structure, including the types and structure of joints, is considered and this is followed by information on the composition, location and functions of muscles, tendons and ligaments. The conformation of every individual horse is determined by his skeletal make-up and musculature. The various points of conformation and the effects they may have upon a horse's soundness and way of going are discussed.

The nervous and sensory systems of sight, smell, hearing, taste and touch control the horse's perceptions of and reactions to his environment. The structures, functions and disorders of these systems are therefore covered. Included in the same section of the book is information on the endocrine system —

the glands and their hormones — since these work in collaboration with the nervous system.

The structures and functions of the circulatory system are explained in a section which includes information on the composition of blood. Disorders such as anaemia and shock are included in this section, as are those circulatory disorders which arise from metabolic imbalance. The closely associated lymphatic system is also described at this point.

In addition to dealing with structure, functions and disorders, the section on the respiratory system includes analysis of the effects of work upon it. Discussion of the urinary system concludes this section of the book.

Within the section entitled 'The Sick Horse', external causes of physiological malfunction are discussed. This section includes information on bacteria and viruses, the body's own defence mechanisms, and the principles of vaccination. Different types of drug used in the treatment of injury and disease are covered, as are further causes of disease, such as poisoning. The book concludes with descriptions of notifiable diseases.

1

SKELETAL STRUCTURE OF THE HORSE

A horse's soundness and his ability to perform satisfactorily, whether in a working role or in the different competitive disciplines, is directly affected by his conformation. It is therefore most important that anyone riding, training or looking after performance horses has a knowledge of both external and internal equine structures and the way in which they contribute to both the static and dynamic conformation of the horse. Knowledge of the horse's skeletal structure and musculature is invaluable when considering aspects of conformation and movement and, coupled with an understanding of the positions and functions of the different tendons and ligaments, will assist greatly in the recognition and diagnosis of lameness. The functions of the skeleton are:

To provide a framework for other body tissues to build upon.

To protect vital organs such as the brain, spinal cord, heart, lungs and kidneys.

To act as a storehouse for calcium and phosphorous. An in-foal mare needs large quantities of these minerals to prevent the excessive withdrawal of them from her own skeleton. This store of minerals is constantly changing – either increasing or

1

decreasing according to nutritional supply and physiological demand. Bones lacking the necessary minerals will become porous and therefore lack strength.

To produce red and white blood cells in certain bones, for example the long bones of the limbs; the ribs; the flat bones of the skull.

To accommodate changing mechanical stresses and the demands of calcium balance, all bones are in a dynamic state of growth and resorbtion throughout life.

The number of bones in the horse's skeleton varies with age as a result of fusion and the conversion of cartilage to bone. However, a normal adult skeleton consists of 205 bones:

The Skull			34
The Spinal Vertebrae:			
Cervical	7		
Thoracic	18		
Lumbar	6		
Sacral	5	(fused)	
Coccygeal	18	(approx.)	54
Ribs and Sternum			37
Forelimbs			40
Hind Limbs			40
			205

BONE STRUCTURE AND COMPOSITION

Bone is a specialized form of connective tissue known as supportive tissue. Other supportive tissues are cartilage, joints, ligaments and tendons. Bone is the hard, rigid form of supportive tissue forming the skeleton of vertebrates. It is composed mainly of inorganic calcium salts, primarily calcium phosphate and calcium carbonate. The organic matter of bone is a collagen-like substance called oissein. In the young horse the proportion

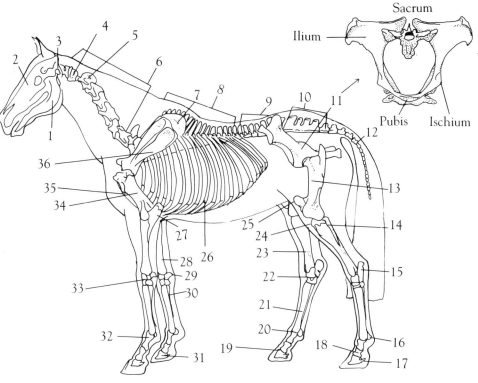

Figure 1 The skeleton of the horse

1. Mandible (lower jaw)
2. Skull
3. Occipital bone
4. Atlas
5. Axis
6. Cervical vertebrae (7)
7. Cartilage of prolongation
8. Thoracic vertebrae (18)
9. Lumbar vertebrae (6)
10. Sacral vertebrae (5)
11. Pelvis (ilium, ischium and pubis)
12. Coccygeal vertebrae (15–20)
13. Femur
14. Fibula
15. Os calcis
16. Sesamoid bones
17. Navicular bone
18. Short pastern bone (second phalanx)
19. Coffin or pedal joint
20. Fetlock joint
21. Cannon bone
22. Tarsus (hock joint)
23. Tibia
24. Stifle joint
25. Patella
26. Ribs; 18 pairs (19 pairs in Arabs)
27. Ulna
28. Radius
29. Pisiform
30. Splint bones
31. Pedal bone (third phalanx)
32. Long pastern bone (first phalanx)
33. Carpus (knee)
34. Humerus
35. Sternum
36. Scapula (shoulder blade)

of organic matter is high, approximately 60 per cent, whereas in the older horse the bones become more brittle and the organic content is reduced to approximately 35 per cent.

Bone is a living tissue and is very responsive to environmental changes, such as changes in physical loading, blood supply and nutrition. Bones can demineralize (therefore becoming less dense) as a result of constant and excessive pressure and increase in size (hypertrophy) as a response to concussion, a process which can be seen in bony enlargements such as splints, bone spavins, etc.

Short bones, and the ends of long bones, produce red and white blood corpuscles. Short bones have red bone marrow in their cavities, while the cavities of the long bones are filled by yellow bone marrow and facilitate the storage of fat.

Classification of bone

Long bones. Include the bones of the limbs. Each has an enlarged end known as an epiphysis which provides a greater bearing surface for the joint, rendering it less liable to dislocation. Bony projections close to the articular enlargements act as attachment sites for muscles, tendons and ligaments.

Short bones. Include the carpal and tarsal bones, os calcis (point of hock), sesamoids, patella. When found on a joint, they act as shock absorbers, for example the small bones of the knee and hock.

Flat bones. Include the cranial plates and scapula. They protect underlying organs.

Irregular bones. Include the bones of the pelvis and the vertebral column. They have a large number of projections for muscle and tendon attachment. Any bone which does not fall into the other three categories is classified as an irregular bone.

Bone formation in the unborn foal

All bone is formed in two steps:

1) Matrix formation. Osteoblasts (bone-producing cells) lay down a calcifiable matrix of a ground substance and fibres called osteoid.

2) Mineralization. Calcium hydroxyapatite crystals are laid down using collagen fibres as a model.

These processes occur by two means:

Membranous ossification

There is no pre-existing cartilage model when, in early intra-uterine life (within the uterus), the bones of the skull and face are formed. At the point in the membrane where the bone is to form (the skull and face), the area is very richly supplied by blood vessels.

The embryonic network of connective tissue is known as mesenchyme and it is the mesenchymal cells which proliferate, some becoming bone-forming cells known as osteoblasts. Certain of these osteoblasts secrete an intercellular substance with which they surround themselves and become calcified, forming mature cells known as osteocytes.

As this process continues spikes of bone are formed, radiating outwards to form a latticework of cancellous (spongy) bone. The spaces between the spikes are gradually filled, forming wide, flat bones which spread out but do not get any thicker.

At birth, the cranial plates are simple plates of cancellous bone but the outer layer, the periosteum, lays down dense or compact bone on the top and bottom to form tables. These tables are held together at birth by connective tissue called sutures, which fuse in adult life.

Membranous ossification also enlarges the width of the long bones.

Cartilaginous ossification

This occurs in all of the long bones of the body, and starts slightly later in intrauterine life than membranous ossification. A long bone forms from a cartilaginous shape known as a model, which has four limb buds. The first changes occur in the mesenchyme cells in the middle of the shaft of the model.

The cells start to proliferate, become condensed and form a rough outline of the shape of the bone to be.

At the central core these mesenchymal cells differentiate into cartilage-forming cells (chondroblasts), which secrete an intercellular substance (ICS) which pushes the cells apart, resulting in a clear cartilaginous model of the future bone.

The chondroblasts then become full cartilage cells (chondrocytes) which mature in the mid-section of the shaft, while the ends and sides of the model grow longer and wider. As the chondrocytes reach a certain size they secrete phosphatase, which activates the process of calcification. Once this process is complete no nutrients can pass through, so the chondrocytes die.

As a result of the increased development of the embryo's vascular system, the cells of the outer cartilaginous shell (perichondrium) go through a series of changes to become bone-forming cells (osteoblasts), which lay down a thin shell of bone and mature into osteocytes. As bone is now formed the perichondrium becomes membranous, at which stage it is known as the periosteum. This will provide a means of attachment for ligaments and tendons, produce new bone from its lining of osteoblasts and bring nutrients to the bone.

Bone is being continually laid down forming a latticework of cancellous bone which has cartilage inside. The cartilage matures and forms bone which, combined with that formed by the osteogenic cells of the periosteum, helps to strengthen the shaft. Once the shaft is strong, the cancellous bone is no longer needed and is reabsorbed, leaving a space known as the marrow cavity.

Secondary centres of ossification appear later. These are known as the epiphyseal centres of ossification and occur in the cartilage of the expanded ends, with bone being laid down and the width increasing.

Some cartilage remains and becomes the articular surface of the bone. The epiphyseal disc or plate separates the diaphysis (shaft) from the epiphysis (articular enlargement). See Figure 2. Growth through the epiphyseal plates carries on through life until cartilage cells stop multiplying and fusion of the epiphysis and diaphysis occurs. Timing of this varies in the individual bones, examples being as follows:

Age at which Epiphyseal Plates Close

	Long Pastern	Cannon Bone	Tibia
Proximal (Upper End)	6—15 months	Before birth	36—42 months
Distal (Lower End)	1 month	6—18 months	17—24 months

With the exception of the articular ends, all bone is covered by periosteum. Within this membrane coarse, collagenous fibres known as 'Sharpey's fibres' form. Their functions are to attach the periosteum to the bone and to attach tendons to bone.

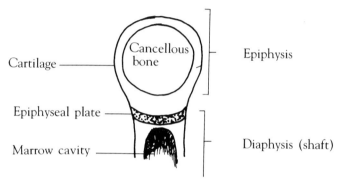

Figure 2 Structure of a long bone

Structure of compact (dense) bone

The outer bone which forms the shaft of long bones is very dense, so is called compact bone. The interior bone is cancellous (spongy). Bone exists in two main forms — woven and lamellar.

Woven bone is the first-produced immature form and is characterized by random (woven) organization of its fibrous elements. During development, woven bone is remodelled to form lamellar bone.

Lamellar bone is composed of successive layers, each of which has a highly organized structure. Lamellar bone may be compact or cancellous.

Compact bone is composed of parallel columns made of concentric bony layers (lamellae) arranged around a central tunnel containing blood and lymphatic vessels and nerves. The central tunnel and layers of bone are known as a Haversian system. The columns are arranged parallel to the long axis of the bone.

Each Haversian system begins as a broad channel made by the burrowing activity of bone resorbing cells; osteoclasts. Osteoblasts (bone-producing cells) then lay down lamellae of bone, gradually decreasing the diameter of the Haversian canal. Eventually the osteoblasts become trapped as osteocytes in the bone matrix.

At the outermost aspect of compact bone, Haversian systems give way to concentric lamellae of dense bone, laid down at the bone surface by osteoblasts of the periosteum. Towards the centre, similar but irregular lamellae merge with spikules of spongy bone.

The Haversian systems are linked to each other and to the marrow through horizontal canals known as Volkmann's canals. These canals also bring nutrients to the bone from the periosteum.

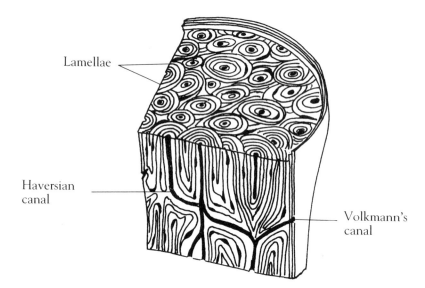

Figure 3 Section of long bone showing Haversian systems and Volmann's canals

MAJOR BONE GROUPS

The skull

The many bones of the skull are fused together to form immovable joints; skull sutures. The skull consists of two main parts; the cranium, which houses and protects the brain, and the face, which encloses the nasal and oral cavities.

The cranial cavity is partially divided by a bony partition, the internal occipital protuberance. The front houses the fore brain and the rear houses the hind brain. The spinal cord lies in the spinal canal and continues into the hind brain through an opening in the skull known as the foramen magnum.

Within the nasal cavity are the turbinate bones (nasal conchae) which are covered with a mucus-secreting tissue, epithelium, which warms, moistens and filters the inspired (incoming) air.

Within the oral cavity the front part of the roof of the mouth is known as the hard palate, and the rear part as the soft palate. The soft palate separates the oral cavity from the pharynx. On the floor of the mouth lies the tongue, a mass of muscle which is attached to the hyoid bone.

The sinuses and guttural pouch

Because the horse has evolved as a grazing animal he requires large, powerful jaws and teeth to keep pace with the continual process of mastication. The mandible, or lower jawbone is large enough to accommodate the molars easily. However, in order to house the jaws and teeth, the bones of the skull need to offer a wide and strong surface area — if this were achieved through bone deposition the head would weigh far too much. The skull is, therefore, widened and strengthened with air-filled cavities known as sinuses. The sinuses, although not involved with the sense of smell, are lined by a continuation of the nasal membrane and are affected when a horse suffers from a nasal infection. Also, although they are not directly involved in respiratory air flow, during expiration the air within the sinuses is partially exchanged.

Each side of the head accommodates several sinuses:

The frontal sinus extends from the upper part of the nasal bones and lies beneath the lower part of the forehead. This sinus allows for widening of the skull without extra weight — as a result of this widening, the eyes are positioned in a lateral manner, giving a wide field of vision which is essential for survival. The frontal sinus also enables the head to carry a wider upper jaw, offering sufficient space for teeth and nasal passages. The position of this sinus offers protection to the brain. The sinus is in two halves, each separated by a thin bony partition and each connected to the large superior maxillary sinus.

The superior maxillary sinus extends beneath the orbit (eye socket) and downwards towards the molar teeth. The roots of the last three molars protrude into this airspace, therefore any infection or injury to those teeth could result in an infection of the sinus.

The inferior maxillary sinus is separated from the superior by a plate of bone. This smaller airspace also communicates directly with the nasal cavity.

The sphenopalatine sinus lies below the ethmoid bones and is divided into two areas: the sphenoid sinus is to the back of the head whilst in front lies the palatine sinus, which is connected to the superior maxillary sinus. Should the sphenoid sinus become infected, its position makes it difficult to drain.

The guttural pouch is a cavity which extends back under the atlas and forwards over the opening of the throat (see Figure 4). The eustachian tube connects the middle ear with the throat, with the guttural pouch extending over the tissues surrounding the throat. Infection within this pouch can present severe problems as many important nerves and blood vessels run through or close to it. The most common disease of the guttural pouch is called guttural pouch mycosis — a fungal infection within

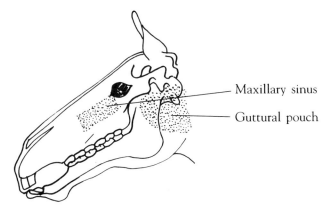

Maxillary sinus

Guttural pouch

Figure 4 The maxillary sinus and guttural pouch

the pouch. The most common sign is spontaneous epistaxis (nosebleed) caused by damage of the internal carotid artery by the fungus (see Chapter 6). A number of nerve paralyses may also occur, as nerves supplying the throat, eyelids and tongue pass in close vicinity to the guttural pouch.

The vertebral column

The vertebral column is commonly known as the spine. Its functions are:

To provide strength for the suspension and propulsion of the bodyweight.

To provide an attachment for the ribs which protect the organs within the thoracic cavity.

To protect the spinal cord.

The spine consists of a string of incompressible bony vertebrae which articulate with each other. Between each is a slightly compressible cartilaginous disc. There are, however, no discs in the spaces between the joints of the atlas and axis. The intervertebral discs consist of dense fibrous tissue. They act as shock absorbers and allow a certain amount of movement along the spine.

The spinal column is divided, for reference, into the following groups of vertebrae:

Cervical. The first two cervical vertebrae are the atlas and axis. There are five other cervical vertebrae, all of which have reduced spinous processes to allow for the wide range of movement required by the neck.

Thoracic. The ribs encircle the chest from sternum to spine attaching to the thoracic vertebrae which are capable of only limited movement. There are eighteen pairs of ribs; the first eight pairs attach directly to the sternum. These are known as 'true' ribs. The other ten pairs attach to the sternum by means of cartilaginous extensions and are known as 'false' ribs.

Lumbar. The loin muscles attach to the lumbar vertebrae which have very rigid, well defined processes. The forward thrust of the hind legs is transferred to the body through the lumbar vertebrae, which are large and stout.

Sacral. The five sacral vertebrae are fused together forming the sacrum. The sacrosciatic ligament extends from the sacrum and coccygeal bones to the pelvic bone below. The upper part of the ilium meets the sacrum, forming the sacroiliac joints which have a basic capacity for shock absorption.

Coccygeal. The coccygeal vertebrae form the tail. They are small and have very reduced processes as they are not subjected to any strong muscular tensions.

The foreleg

Although the foreleg supports two-thirds of the bodyweight the scapula (shoulder blade) is free from any bony connection with the rest of the body. However, because it is attached to the trunk by muscles, the scapula is capable of extensive movements. The main muscle of attachment is the ventral serrate muscle. The way in which this and other muscles are attached between the scapula and the trunk provides a means of shock absorption.

The scapula slopes down and forward to meet the humerus which then slopes back and down to the elbow, meeting the radius and reduced ulna which are fused together. The ulna has a blunt rearward projection called the oleocranon (point of elbow).

The carpus or knee corresponds to the wrist of man and contains seven bones. The small bones are arranged in two rows with the pisiform or accessory carpal bone projecting at the rear. Below the knee is the large metacarpal or cannon bone, a long bone with a rounded shaft. The front surface is smooth and convex, the rear surface slightly flattened, with roughened edges on the outer and inner aspects for attachment of the two small metacarpal (splint) bones. The lower extremities end at the lower third of the large metacarpal in a small, bulbous point called the button. In the young horse there is slight mobility between the metacarpal bones. As the horse matures, they become ossified. Over-stimulation of bone growth, for example as caused by hard work on hard ground will, particularly with young horses, cause exostosis – increased growth of bone. When this affects the fusion of the metacarpus the resulting bony enlargement is known as a splint.

The first phalanx or long pastern bone has a cylindrical shaft, the surfaces of which are roughened to accommodate ligamentous insertions. The upper end articulates with the large metacarpal bone to form the fetlock joint. At the rear of this joint is a pair of small pyramidal bones, the sesamoids. These bones are attached strongly to the first phalanx and quite weakly to the suspensory ligament. The lower surface of the first phalanx articulates with the second phalanx or short pastern bone, forming the pastern joint. The second phalanx is cube-shaped with roughened surfaces to allow the attachment of ligaments and the superficial flexor tendon. The surface of the second phalanx meets the third phalanx (pedal or coffin bone) to form the coffin joint. There is a sesamoid bone called the navicular bone behind the coffin joint. This is a small, trans-versely elongated bone, the function of which is to reinforce the joint when the foot strikes the ground. The shape of the third phalanx corresponds with the shape of the hoof.

The anatomy of the foot is discussed further in another book in this series: *The Horse: The Foot, Shoeing and Lameness.*

The hind leg

The pelvic girdle is made up of the fused sacral vertebrae and two hip bones (os coxai). Each hip bone consists of three bones fused together — the ilium, ischium and pubis. The tuber sacrale (point of croup) is on the front of the ilium near the sacrum, while on the outer edge is the tuber coxae (point of hip). The ilium fuses with the ischium at the hip joint. There is a rearward projection on the ischium called the tuber ischii (point of buttock). The lower part of the ischium, along with the pubis, forms the floor of the pelvis.

The angle at which the sacrum lies in relation to the pelvic floor will affect the overall diameter of the inside of the pelvis. Should the sacrum tilt downwards, it may cause difficulties in foaling.

The hind leg attaches to the pelvic girdle in a depression called the acetabulum, into which the ball-like head of the femur fits to form the hip joint.

The femur or thigh bone slopes down and forward to meet the tibia at the stifle. At the front of the stifle joint is a sesamoid bone called the patella which corresponds to the human kneecap. The patella is joined to the tibial tuberosity by the patellar ligaments and is enabled to slide up and down in a groove by activities within the quadriceps femoris muscle group. It is, however, possible for the patella to be displaced from the groove and become locked, thus activating the horse's hind leg locking mechanism.

Beside the tibia is a much reduced fibula which is approximately 10 cm (4 in) long. The tibia slopes down and back towards the hock which contains six bones and corresponds to the human ankle. The tuber calcis (point of hock) projects upwards and backwards. The structure below the hock is similar to that of the foreleg, with the cannon and splint bones being known as the large and small metatarsals.

JOINTS

Joints occur where two or more bones meet. Their type and form is determined by their function and the degree of mobility required. Not all joints are constructed to allow movement, nor are they necessarily permanent.

Joints are divided into four main groups: bony, fibrous, cartilaginous and synovial.

Bony joints are those such as the pelvis, which has three elements fused together — the ilium, ischium and pubis.

Fibrous joints are fixed joints composed of fibrous connective tissue between bones, such as skull sutures.

Cartilaginous joints are divided into primary and secondary cartilaginous joints. Primary joints are those where bony surfaces are united by cartilage, as seen in the epiphyseal plates in long bones before ossification. Secondary cartilaginous joints are united by a fibrocartilaginous disc such as the intervertebral discs. This type of joint provides a resilient bond as is needed in the spine. The movement possible depends upon the thickness of the disc.

Cartilage has a porous nature, resembling a sponge. As it is closely moulded to bone it has no nutrient blood vessels, but receives nutrition from the vascular network in the synovial membrane and blood vessels in the periosteum and marrow cavities. Young cartilage is white and glistening but with age it becomes thinner, firmer and less elastic, with a less regular surface and turns yellow in colour.

Articular cartilage (that which lines joints) is able to withstand great forces of compression because of its wear-resistant, low friction, slightly compressible and elastic surface and, although smooth in appearance it is, in fact, a series of valleys and peaks with synovial fluid trapped in the valleys.

Synovial joints are free-moving joints, the bones of which are linked by a fibrous capsule. The bone ends are covered by cartilage which, aided by synovial fluid, reduces friction.

Synovial fluid is secreted by the synovial membrane. This membrane lines the non-articular part of a synovial joint, and all tendon sheaths. Its surface is lubricated by an eggwhite-like fluid, synovia, which is secreted and absorbed by the membrane. Synovial fluid is a clear, pale yellow, viscous, slightly alkaline fluid containing few cells. Its functions are to provide a liquid environment and nutritive source for the articular cartilage and discs. It also acts as a lubricant and helps to reduce the erosion of joint surfaces. However, the major lubricating shock-absorbing function comes from cartilage itself.

Classification of synovial joints

If a joint has two articular surfaces it is known as a simple joint; if it has more it is known as a compound joint. Joints are also classified as follows:

Hinge joint. This allows a 'to and fro' movement via a convex to concave surface — for example, the pastern joint.

Plane joint. This has fairly flat articular surfaces which give a gliding movement, as found between the articular processes of adjacent vertebrae.

Pivot joint. A peg-like process rotates in a socket allowing a sideways turning, for example the joint between the first two cervical vertebrae, the atlas and axis.

Condylar joint. A knuckle-shaped surface articulates with a deep, cup-shaped cavity, allowing movement in a single plane. An example is the joint between the atlas and occipital bone, which allows the head to nod up and down.

Ball and socket joint. The globular head of one bone fits into the cup-like cavity (acetabulum) of another. For example, the hip joint.

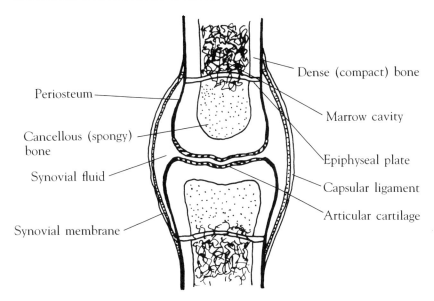

Figure 5 Structure of a simple synovial joint

2

MUSCLES, TENDONS AND LIGAMENTS

Movement is initiated through the combined effect of the activities of skeletal muscle, tendons and ligaments upon the skeleton. Each is a different form of connective tissue with its own distinct function. By contracting, muscles cause movement of bones. The muscles are attached to the bones by tendons. Ligaments connect many of the bones and cartilages to each other.

MUSCLES

Muscles are divided into three main types:

Smooth muscles are involuntary muscles found in the digestive and reproductive tracts, the blood vascular system, bladder and bowels.

Cardiac muscles are specialized muscles found only in the heart.

Skeletal or striated muscles are attached to, support and move the skeleton. It is the skeletal muscles which form the 'meat' of the horse and are responsible for locomotion. It is with these that we are chiefly concerned here.

Skeletal muscles

These muscles are under the voluntary control of the horse and amount to approximately one third of the bodyweight, there being, on average, seven hundred skeletal muscles in the body. The functions of these muscles are:

1) To support the skeletal structure.

2) To move the skeleton through contraction of the muscle fibres.

3) To maintain joint stability, preventing undesirable, excessive movement.

4) Heat production by shivering.

Muscles contract to bring about an action: flexor muscles contract causing the joint to articulate. The joint is then straightened by contraction of the corresponding extensor muscle. It should be noted that extension of a muscle is always a passive process, each muscle group being opposed by another with an antagonistic effect.

Abductor muscles carry the limb away from the mid-line of the body whilst adductor muscles carry the limb towards it.

In order for muscles to perform these functions they have attachments at each end: the origin, which tends to be the less movable part and the insertion, the more movable part. Upon contraction the insertion moves towards the origin. The attachments may be directly onto the skeleton, or via a connection of deep fascia (fibrous tissue).

Composition of skeletal muscle

Muscle fibres

Skeletal muscle is composed of millions of long, slender fibres known as myofibrils. These are built from various proteins, predominantly myosin and actin. Each myofibril is a single cell, elongated and cylindrical. These fibres lie parallel to each other, supported and bound by connective tissue within the muscle belly. This connective tissue binds the muscle fibres to the tendons at either end. When stimulated by a nervous impulse, the myofibrils slide over one another with a ratchet-type mechanism causing the muscle to shorten, thicken and therefore contract — the muscle fibres themselves do not actually shorten.

The contraction of muscles requires a supply of energy. In addition to the myofibrils, muscle contains tiny intracellular organs called mitochondria. These store the carbohydrate energy-giving substance glycogen, which is broken down to release energy through a chemical reaction caused by enzymes, which are also stored within the muscle cells. To fuel this process, oxygen is brought to the muscles by the blood supply and is stored in the red muscle pigment, myoglobin. Myoglobin is a protein which can bind oxygen to itself.

All muscles contain a mix of three types of fibre — slow-twitch, high oxidative fast-twitch and low oxidative fast-twitch. The level of each is often influenced by the horse's breeding and will, in turn, have an effect upon the type of work to which an individual horse is best suited.

Slow-twitch fibres have relatively slow contractions but a great capacity for using oxygen. It is these which are important for endurance work.

High oxidative fast-twitch fibres contain large amounts of myoglobin, which gives the muscle a dark red colour and enables the use of large amounts of oxygen. A preponderance of this type of fibre allows a horse to work at relatively high speed over a distance.

Low oxidative fast-twitch fibres contain much less myoglobin, and are very pale in colour (almost white). Muscle in which these fibres predominate provides powerful acceleration, but fatigues quickly.

Waste products such as lactic acid and carbon dioxide are created as a result of muscular activity. These waste products are removed via the bloodstream. (More information is given further on in this book; Chapter 6 — The Respiratory System.)

Muscle bellies

Muscle bellies (the typical muscle forms) come in various shapes and sizes. Some are flat and sheet-like, for example the latissimus dorsi, external abdominal oblique and trapezius. In these the muscle fibres are long, with flattened tendinous attachments, and offer a wide range of movement.

Long, strap-like muscles such as the brachiocephalic also have long fibres, but the muscles of the forearm and thigh have shorter fibres densely packed in the belly, resulting in great strength. Such muscles are known as pennate muscles.

TENDONS

A tendon is a fibrous cord of connective tissue continuous with the fibres of a muscle, attaching the muscle to bone, cartilage or other muscle. Tendons insert into bone or cartilage by means of small spikules known as 'Sharpey's fibres'. Where a muscle needs a wide area of attachment the tendon spreads out to form an aponeurosis.

Tendons form in the embryo from fibroblasts (fibre-forming cells) which proliferate, becoming tightly packed, as the tendon grows. As development continues, the fibres become arranged in longitudinal rows and secrete collagen, the main supporting protein of connective tissue. The production of collagen is a continuous process — it takes six months to renew completely the collagen within a lower limb tendon. Excess, old or damaged collagen is broken down by enzymes and removed via the bloodstream. The blood supply through tendons is poor and in the event of injury, it becomes disrupted, leading to reduced nutrient and oxygen supply which hampers the healing process.

The fibres of which tendons are composed have a one-directional helical arrangement, with cross-linkages and orderly compartmentalization of bundles. These features are mimicked, but *not* replicated by the scar tissue that forms at the site of tendon repair. Thus, once damaged, a tendon will always be weaker. Also, if the tendon ends are allowed to retract from each other after a serious injury, they will atrophy and be re-sorbed, since tendons do not contain their own cells to initiate repair. Repair processes come from the adjacent soft tissue.

The tendon sheath

Where a tendon is in a position to rub against bone or other hard surfaces, it is enclosed in a sheath. This takes the form of an inner sheath which encloses and is firmly attached to the tendon, and an outer connective tissue tube which is attached to its surrounding surface. The space between the two sheaths is filled with a lubricant similar to synovial fluid.

LIGAMENTS

Ligaments are composed of bands of white and yellow fibrous tissue, the white being inelastic and the yellow, elastic. They are somewhat flexible but tough and unyielding in consistency. Ligaments can be categorized as follows:

Supporting or *suspending*, for example the suspensory ligament.

Annular — broad bands composed of deep fascia which directs the pull on a tendon.

Inter-osseus — ties bones together, for example the pedal and navicular.

Funicular (or cordlike) — holds bones together.

Ligaments help to limit the movement of joints according to their functions, for example the fetlock, pastern and coffin joints have collateral ligaments on their inner and outer aspects to confine movement to forward and backward only. Ligaments attach to the bone through blending with the periosteum. They usually allow a certain amount of movement; the more that is required, the more yellow elastic tissue is present in the ligament. Conversely, those ligaments holding an immovable joint together will be composed only of inelastic white tissue.

Ligaments are poorly supplied with blood but rich in sensory nerves. Because of the poor blood supply they are very slow to heal after injury. Ligaments do not withstand prolonged stretching. If a joint is forced beyond the limitations set by the ligament, then a very painful sprain will occur. However, since ligaments (and muscles) are usually more elastic than the bone to which they are attached, any severe stress is more likely to break the bone than dislocate the joint or tear the ligament.

The tendons and ligaments of the lower limbs are discussed in full detail in another book in this series, *The Horse: The Foot, Shoeing and Lameness*.

Fascia

The skin and underlying parts are connected to each other by a sheet of fibrous tissue called fascia. Fascia is sheet-like and loose, tending to be most prevalent over the neck and trunk. Deep fascia forms relatively thick sheets of dense, fibrous connective tissue which is attached to the skeleton, ligaments and tendons in places and is adherent to many underlying muscles. In the knee and hock, tendons pass through grooves in the bone surface and are held within the groove by deep fascia forming annular ligaments. A sheet of elastic deep fascia forms the abdominal tunic along the trunk which helps the abdominal muscles support the internal organs.

LOCATION AND FUNCTIONS OF MAJOR MUSCLES, TENDONS AND LIGAMENTS

The head and neck

The many muscles in the head are responsible for the various facial expressions and actions of the lips and eyelids. The horse's neck is long to facilitate grazing. The muscles are large and bulky to allow mobility and carriage of the head. The positioning of the head and neck enables the horse to alter his own centre of gravity — lowering the head brings it forward while raising the head moves it backward. The main muscles and ligaments of the head and neck are:

The massetter, the main muscle of the cheek which closes the jaw and causes the grinding action for chewing.

The brachiocephalic, a broad, strap-like muscle which causes head and neck to swing from side to side, pulls the scapula forward (when the horse is working in collection this muscle raises the scapula as the neck is carried higher) and swings the foreleg forwards.

The tendon of the brachiocephalic muscle originates at the base of the skull. The muscle extends down the side of the neck to just below the point of shoulder.

The rhomboideus muscle lies at the top of the neck and assists in pulling the scapula forwards.

The splenius muscle is also at the top of the neck and acts to extend and turn the neck.

The trapezius originates from the occipital bone and attaches to the spines of the seventh cervical and all of the thoracic vertebrae. It lies over the rhomboideus and splenius in a large, flat sheet on either side of the withers and raises the scapula.

The nuchal ligament assists the muscles of the neck in supporting the head.

The shoulder

The horse's forehand plays an extremely important role as main weight bearer, carrying two-thirds of the bodyweight. While a horse is standing still, especially with his head down, the centre of gravity is well forward in the chest region. When the horse moves off, contraction of the ventral serrate and deep pectoral muscles causes the centre of gravity to be moved backwards. The large ventral serrate, the cranial part of the deep pectoral and the rhomboid are muscles which run from the body and attach to the scapula.

The forelimbs have no bony attachment to the axial skeleton. The weight of the trunk is suspended between the scapulae and the forelimbs, stabilized at the shoulder by a series of muscles. The muscles which act as braces on the forelimb include the brachiocephalic, trapezius, latissimus dorsi and pectoral. The supraspinatus muscle originates below the trapezius muscle and attaches at the point of shoulder. It maintains the shoulder in extension. The latissimus dorsi muscles originate at the lower thoracic vertebrae, pass over the upper part of the thorax and attach to the back of the humerus. They operate to pull the foreleg backwards. The triceps and biceps are muscles which extend the elbow.

The foreleg

Muscles of the foreleg

The muscles of the legs are known as pennate muscles. The belly of such a muscle is attached to both sides of a long tendon. The tendon is well embedded into the belly of the muscle and extends down to the knee, fetlock and digital joints. The fibres of the pennate muscles are short and densely packed, making them very strong. Their tendons run in grooves in the bone across the knee and fetlock and are held in position by condensed deep fascia known as annular ligament.

The radial carpal extensor muscle and tendon is responsible for straightening the knee joint, while the tendons of the lateral carpal flexor muscle cause the knee to flex.

Tendons of the lower leg

Extending downwards from their corresponding muscles are four tendons in the lower foreleg — two extensors on the front and two flexors on the back (see Figure 6.) They are:

The common digital extensor tendon (CDET). This tendon is attached to all of the bones in the foot except the navicular. It runs down the front of the cannon bone and over the fetlock joint towards the lower end of the long pastern bone. Here the tendon receives reinforcement on either side from extensor branches of the suspensory ligament, which increase its width, enabling it to pass over the pastern joint, the short pastern bone, the pedal (coffin) joint and attach to the upper aspect of the pointed centre of the pedal bone (the extensor process). It is held in position by the bands from the suspensory ligament and by ligaments originating from the lower end of the long pastern bone.

The function of the CDET is to extend the bones of the foot and lift the toe.

The lateral digital extensor tendon (LDET). The LDE muscle lies behind the common digital extensor muscle. The tendons of these muscles run down in close contact with each other, the lateral digital extensor lying to the rear of the other and inserting into the outer side of the long pastern bone.

Working in conjunction with the CDET, the function of the LDET is to help extend the bones of the foot.

The deep digital flexor tendon (DDFT). The muscle of this tendon originates at the ulna. The DDFT passes over the back of the knee in the carpal canal and is held in position by a carpal check ligament. It then extends down the back of the cannon bone between the superficial digital flexor tendon and the suspensory ligament. In the middle of the cannon bone the DDFT is joined by the carpal check ligament, known as the inferior check ligament. The tendon then passes over the sesamoid bones, sliding on a glistening pad formed by the inter-sesamoidean ligament, before passing between the two extensions of the superficial digital flexor tendon. At this point the DDFT becomes broad and fanlike, passing over the navicular bone before inserting into the lower surface of the pedal bone.

The superficial digital flexor tendon (SDFT). This tendon passes down the back of the distal humerus where it receives the superior check ligament. It then passes down the back of the cannon bone, completely covering the DDFT. At the lower end of the cannon bone the SDFT widens and encircles the DDFT, forming a ring known as the pastern annular ligament of the fetlock joint, extensions from which then attach to the short and long pastern bones.

The superficial and deep flexor tendons extend down from their muscles in the forearm through to the foot, providing weight-bearing support and preventing the overextension of the fetlock joint (a role in which they are assisted by their check ligaments). Their other chief function, when the horse is in motion, is to flex the joints of the lower leg.

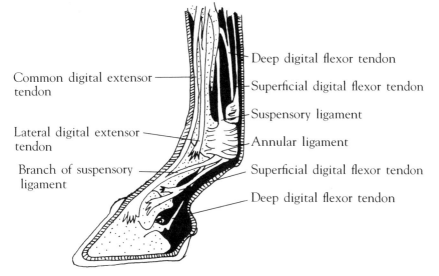

Common digital extensor tendon

Lateral digital extensor tendon

Branch of suspensory ligament

Deep digital flexor tendon

Superficial digital flexor tendon

Suspensory ligament

Annular ligament

Superficial digital flexor tendon

Deep digital flexor tendon

Figure 6 The tendons and ligaments of the lower leg

Ligaments of the lower leg

The suspensory ligament. This lies between the two splint bones close to the back of the cannon bone, originating close to the knee and descending towards the fetlock joint, above which it divides into two branches. Each branch attaches to the corresponding sesamoid bone while some fibres blend in with the common digital extensor tendon. The suspensory ligament provides a form of support for the fetlock joint, preventing it from extending downward too far towards the ground, which would increase the risk of strains.

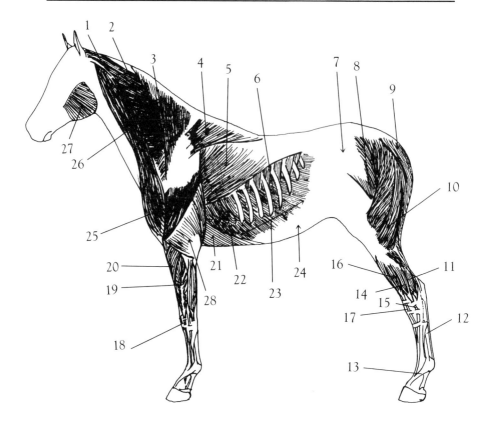

Figure 7 The main superficial muscles

1. Cervical part of rhomboid
2. Splenius
3. Cervical part of trapezius
4. Thoracic part of trapezius
5. Latissimus dorsi
6. External intercostal muscles
7. Gluteal fascia
8. Superficial gluteal muscle
9. Semitendinosus
10. Biceps femoris
11. Deep digital flexor muscle
12. Deep digital flexor tendon
13. Extensor branch of suspensory ligament
14. Lateral digital extensor muscle
15. Lateral digital extensor tendon
16. Long digital extensor muscle
17. Long digital extensor tendon
18. Common digital extensor tendon
19. Common digital extensor muscle
20. Radial carpal extensor muscle
21. Caudal deep pectoral muscle
22. Thoracic part of ventral serrate
23. External abdominal oblique muscles
24. Tendon of external abdominal oblique muscles
25. Deltoid muscle
26. Brachiocephalic
27. Masseter
28. Triceps

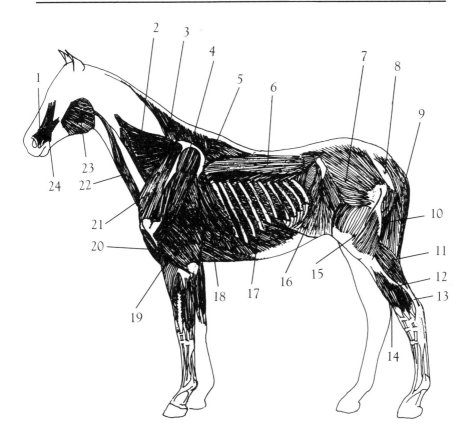

Figure 8 The main deep muscles

1. Lateral nostril dilator
2. Cervical part of ventral serrate
3. Rhomboid muscle
4. Infraspinatus muscle
5. Spinalis dorsi
6. Longissimus dorsi
7. Gluteal muscle
8. Sacrosciatic ligament
9. Semitendinosus
10. Semimembranosus
11. Gastrocnemius
12. Soleus
13. Achilles' tendon
14. Peroneus tertius
15. Lateral vastus muscle
16. Internal abdominal oblique muscles
17. External abdominal oblique muscles
18. Thoracic part of ventral serrate
19. Triceps
20. Biceps
21. Supraspinatus
22. Sternocephalic
23. Masseter
24. Levator muscle of upper lip

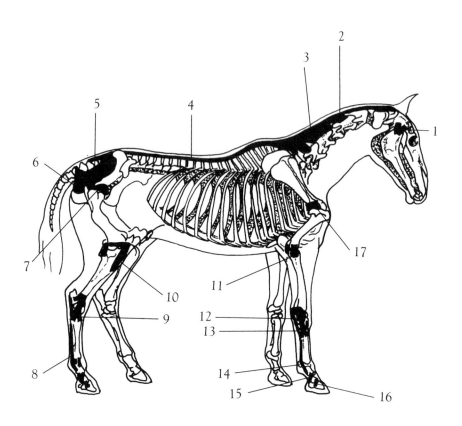

Figure 9 The major ligaments

1. Caudal ligament of jaw joint
2. Funicular part of nuchal ligament
3. Lamellar part of nuchal ligament
4. Supraspinous ligament
5. Sacroiliac ligament
6. Sacrosciatic ligament
7. Capsular ligament of hip joint
8. Suspensory ligament
9. Collateral ligament of tarsal joint
10. Patellar ligaments
11. Collateral ligament of elbow joint
12. Collateral ligament of carpal joint
13. Distal ligament of accessory carpal bone
14. Collateral sesamoidean ligament
15. Collateral ligament of pastern joint
16. Collateral ligament of coffin joint
17. Capsular ligament of shoulder joint

Check ligaments. The inferior check ligament is below the knee. Its functions are to prevent undue strain being applied to the flexor tendons and to assist in supporting the horse, thus allowing him to sleep whilst standing. This ligament is connected to the deep flexor tendon. The superior check ligament is above the knee and connects to the superficial flexor tendon at the back of the humerus. It acts to assist the inferior check ligament.

The anatomy of the lower leg is discussed in greater depth in another book in this series, *The Horse: The Foot, Shoeing and Lameness.*

The trunk

Muscles of the trunk

The spinalis dorsi muscle lies beneath the thoracic part of the trapezius, either side of the withers.

The longissimus dorsi, otherwise known as the lumbar muscles, extend back from the spinalis dorsi.

The external abdominal oblique muscles help support the weight of the internal organs and raise the floor of the abdomen to help with processes such as urination, defecation, foaling and expiration.

The internal abdominal oblique muscles lie beneath the external ones.

The internal and external intercostal muscles are respectively the deep and superficial muscles found between the ribs.

Ligaments of the spine

The muscle groups around the spine are designed to support the spine in conjunction with the abdominal muscles and three important ligaments. These ligaments, attached to the vertebrae along the length of the spine, are:

The ventral ligament, which lies on the underside of the vertebrae.

The dorsal ligament, which forms the floor of the spinal cord.

The supraspinous ligament, which attaches at the poll and extends down to the sacrum. In the withers and neck area fanlike extensions reach down and attach to the spines of the cervical vertebrae. In this area the ligament is known as the nuchal ligament. It helps to support the head and neck whilst maintaining a traction force to the spine which assists with support, particularly in the potentially weak thoraco-lumbar area.

Additionally, the lumbodorsal fascia attaches to the spinous processes of the thoracic and lumbar vertebrae and forms the tendon of origin of the chest and abdominal muscles.

The hindquarters

The superficial gluteal muscle, attached by gluteal fascia to the sacrum, helps maintain the hip joint in extension.

The biceps femoris, semitendinosus and semimembranosus are the three muscles which make up the hamstring group. The biceps femoris is the largest of the three and helps maintain the hip joint in extension. The tarsal tendon extends down from this group.

The gastrocnemius extends from the rear of the femur, down the back of the gaskin to the point of hock. This muscle is closely associated with the superficial digital flexor muscle which attaches at the point of hock and assists in maintaining the hock in extension, taking some of the strain off the gastrocnemius.

The soleus is closely associated with the gastrocnemius, to form part of the triceps surae group.

The peroneus tertius extends from the femur to the cannon bone and, when working in opposition to the superficial digital muscle, causes the stifle and hock joints to move.

The long digital extensor muscle originates at the lower end of the femur. Its tendon passes over the front of the hock. Below the hock, this tendon is joined by the LDET to form the CDET, which inserts at the highest point of the extensor process of the pedal bone.

The Achilles' tendon, one of the largest tendons in the body, extends down from the soleus and gastrocnemius muscles over the point of hock.

The sacrosciatic ligament extends from the sacrum and coccygeal vertebrae down to the pelvic bone, forming the basis of the pelvic walls. This ligament is in the form of a sheet which fuses with part of the hamstring group.

Other than the above, the arrangements of tendons and ligaments correspond with those of the lower foreleg.

The hind leg locking mechanism

The horse, while standing, is able to operate a hind leg locking system to alleviate muscular fatigue. The system works as follows. The patella is attached to the tibial tuberosity by the three patellar ligaments. In order to lock the hind leg, the patella is raised and hooked over the top of the enlarged upper end of the trochlear ridge of the femur. The system is unlocked by contraction of the quadriceps femoris and the biceps femoris, which action lifts the patella off the ridge.

3

CONFORMATION

Conformation is the result of the horse's skeletal make-up and musculature. When assessing a horse's conformation and suitability to perform a specific task, perhaps with a view to purchase, there are many points to look for.

OVERALL IMPRESSION

Bring the horse out of the stable, stand back and look at him as a whole. Start with the 'three Ps':

Proportion – the horse should generally appear to be 'in proportion'; the front should match the hindquarters.

Performance – what is he required to do? He must be tough and sound enough to maintain the level of work necessary.

·Paces – how will his conformation affect his movement?

Bear in mind his age and stage of training, whether stabled or grass kept, whether it is a freezing cold day or extremely hot. These points may affect his appearance. Try to recognize the basic skeletal structure and take into account any circumstances which may affect muscle, skin and coat. If possible, find out the current workload of the horse. For example, the physique of a fit eventer will differ from that of a broodmare.

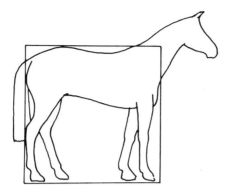

Figure 10 A well proportioned horse

SPECIFIC FEATURES

The overall impression is the sum product of various individual features, each with its own significance.

The head

This should be in proportion to the body. A convex profile (Roman nose) is an indication of slightly common breeding and is generally associated with a good temperament and genuine nature. However, the forehead should not be convex as this often indicates a difficult temperament. A concave profile — a dished face — may be a sign of Arab blood found in more finely bred animals.

The ears of a show animal should be small and neat. Long ears are often a sign of good speed, courage and honesty.

The eyes should be large, clear and prominent. Small 'piggy' eyes, particularly showing a lot of white, may indicate a less than genuine nature. However, the *expression* in the eyes is the best guide to the horse's nature. 'Wall eyes' are blue for genetic reasons. Similarly, albino or cream animals often have pink eyes, which are not really indicative of their temperament.

The nostrils must be wide to allow a good air intake.

The upper and lower jaws should meet evenly. If the upper jaw is too long it is known as a 'sow' or 'parrot mouth'. Both conditions can cause problems when biting grass and, because of the irregular wearing of the teeth, it can be difficult to age the horse accurately.

An important point affecting head carriage and performance is that of the thickness around the jowl region and how the head is set on the neck. There should be room to admit two fingers' width between the lower aspect of the top bone of the neck (the atlas) and the lower jaw (mandible) when the head is raised. Ideally the jaw must not be too thick or fleshy because this may affect the horse's ability to flex correctly at the poll. There should be at least one hand's width between the mandibles at the throat — a smaller gap has been associated with roaring.

The neck

The length of the neck must be relative to the size of the horse. It should not appear to come out too low down between the shoulders as this would put the horse naturally onto the forehand.

A very thick 'bull' neck can give a strong ride and make it difficult to achieve lightness and balance. When the topline muscles, the trapezius and rhomboid, are underdeveloped, a 'ewe neck' results. A ewe neck caused purely by poor muscular development can be resolved by remedial schooling. The real problem ewe neck is that caused by the set on of the neck and the arrangement of the cervical vertebrae. A ewe-necked horse will carry his head high and find it extremely difficult to work in a rounded outline. A constantly high head carriage may cause the muscles of the underside of the neck, the sterno-cephalic, to become overdeveloped.

A young and/or unschooled horse may lack muscle over the topline, but this is not a conformation fault. However, there should be an unbroken curve from poll to withers which will increase and develop as the horse's training progresses.

The chest

Look at the chest from the front. If both forelegs appear to 'come out of the same hole' there may be a tendency to brush.

The chest should be reasonably broad and muscular. However,

a chest that is too broad will give a 'rolling' sort of stride and may make lateral work difficult.

The withers and shoulder

The ideal wither is well defined but not too prominent. A flat or very high, bony wither causes problems when trying to fit a saddle. Horses who are very overweight may have ill-defined withers.

The ideal shoulder is well muscled without being too heavy, that is, 'loaded'. The angle at which the scapula lies gives the slope of shoulder. An upright shoulder is prone to jarring, so the limb is more susceptible to concussion-related conditions. The stride will be relatively short and difficulty may be experienced with extended work. A sloping shoulder gives a more springy ride and allows the horse to take longer strides. A very small shoulder will restrict movement, while a very large one may lead to a lack of nimbleness, particularly when jumping combination obstacles.

The back, trunk and loins

A short back is stronger, though less flexible, than a long one. The latter may give a very comfortable ride and many horses who gallop well have long backs. To ensure strength the horse must be 'well ribbed up' that is, the last rib must be no more than 50 mm (2 in) away from the point of hip.

The ribs must be 'well sprung' and deep through the girth to provide good heart and lung room as opposed to being flat and 'slab-sided'. The back may have a slight dip in it but an exaggerated dip, known as a 'hollow' or 'sway' back, will present problems with saddle fitting. An exaggerated upward curve of the spine is known as a 'roach back', and can also make saddle fitting difficult.

A 'herring-gutted' horse has an upward slope from front to back on the underline of the belly. This can cause the girth and saddle to slip backwards, so necessitates a hunting-style breastplate. If this upward slope is particularly exaggerated around the flanks the horse is described as being 'tucked up'.

This is normally an indication of stress, perhaps as a result of overexertion, illness or cold as opposed to a permanent conformation defect. A horse who is generally looking lean through hard work, training or lack of food is said to have 'run up light'. This can generally be corrected by rest and good food.

The loins must be short and well muscled for strength because the lumbar vertebrae do not gain any support from the ribs, even though it is these which transfer the thrust from the hind limbs to the body.

The hindquarters

The hindquarters must be well muscled with good length from the point of hip to hock. 'Well let down' hocks are often indicative of good speed.

A horse with his croup higher than his withers, sometimes called a 'jumper's bump', has a tendency to be thrown naturally onto the forehand and may find collected work difficult. Many youngsters are 'croup high' but once a horse is mature the withers should be higher than the croup. The croup-high horse will need particularly strong, sound forelimbs and feet to cope with the extra weight borne by the forehand.

A 'goose rump' describes quarters that droop downwards from the croup to a tail set down low.

When viewed from behind there must be a good width between the hips, which must also be level.

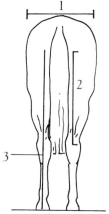

1. Good width between hips
2. 'Well let down' hocks
3. Straight limb

Figure 11 View of well proportioned hindquarters

The forelegs

The conformation of the forelegs will probably be one of the greatest influences on the horse's future soundness. Most lameness in competition horses occurs in the forelegs as a result of strain imposed when landing over fences and from galloping, particularly when the going is hard or uneven. The better the foreleg conformation, the better are the chances of the horse remaining sound.

There must be room at the elbow to allow for movement; particularly important when working in extension. The forearm must be well muscled with good length for speed.

Figure 12 shows a vertical line (A) extending downwards from the point of shoulder passing through the centre of the forearm, knee, cannon bone, fetlock and foot. This ensures regular, even weight distribution and wear on the feet, all joints, tendons and muscles.

The knees must be broad and flat in front to allow room for the collection of small bones and ligaments. They should be relatively deep from front to back. Shallowness here is termed 'calf kneed'. When viewed from the side, the knee joint should appear straight.

Figure 13 shows vertical lines (B) extending downward from the centre of suspension of the forelimb to the centre of the

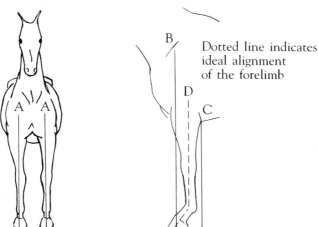

Dotted line indicates
ideal alignment
of the forelimb

**Figure 12 View of a well
proportioned forehand**

**Figure 13 Side view of a foreleg,
showing good alignment**

foot and (C) from the point of elbow to the ground. These help in assessing the straightness of the limb. Should the knee protrude forwards over toward line (B), it is known as being 'over at the knee' and is unacceptable in show classes although this condition does not put excessive strain on the tendons. The opposite condition ('back at the knee'), whereby the knee extends backwards causing a concave line in front of itself, is more serious as extra strain is placed on the tendons and excessive forces are exerted on the dorsal (front) aspects of the knee bones, predisposing them to 'slab' or 'chip' fractures.

The measurement taken around the cannon bone and tendons just below the knee is used to determine the amount of 'bone'. The amount of bone should be in relation to the type and stamp of horse. As an approximate guide a lightweight 16.2 hh horse should have at least 20 cm (8 in) bone. The cannon bone should not be overlong. If it is relatively short it, and its associated tendons, will be stronger. If the measurement just below the knee is less than that further down the cannon bone, ('tied in below the knee'), this may restrict the action of the tendons.

The fetlocks must be large enough to allow room for joint movement and should give an impression of flatness rather than roundness. The pasterns should not be too long and sloping as this exerts greater strain on the fetlock joint and tendons. However, a short, upright pastern increases jarring so may lead to concussion-related ailments.

The hind legs

The thighs should be well muscled and hocks 'well let down'. When viewing from behind, imagine a vertical line extending downward from the point of buttock to the ground. This line must pass through the centre at the hock, cannon bone, fetlock and foot. (See Figure 11, line 3). Hocks which turn inward away from these vertical lines are called 'cow hocks'. The opposite condition is known as being 'bow hocked'. Again, these conditions can cause uneven wear on joints, tendons and feet. Hocks should be large and square-shaped to allow room for bones, tendons and ligaments.

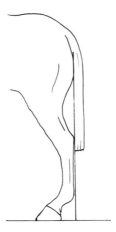

Figure 14 Side view of a hind leg, showing good alignment

When viewed from the side, a vertical line extending down-ward from the point of buttock to the ground (see Figure 14) will help to assess the correct alignment of the hind leg. If the limb appears to be behind this line, the horse is likely to be fast but will find collected work more difficult. If the hocks are forward of this line it improves the horse's balance, but probably means less speed. If the hocks are well forward of this line with a concave line in front of the hock and a slant to the cannon bone, it is a weakness known as 'sickle-hocked'.

The feet

While a horse is standing and moving at leisure, the forefeet bear approximately 60 per cent of the horse's bodyweight. On landing over a fence, one forelimb will bear all of the bodyweight momentarily. Boxy, upright feet will be prone to jarring while large, flat feet may be more susceptible to corns and bruising of the sole. The forefeet should be rounded and a pair. When viewed from the side, the slope of the hoof wall should be continuous with that of the pastern as shown by the dotted line (D) in Figure 13. When viewed from the front, the feet should face forwards. Toes which turn in are known as 'pigeon toes'. This fault causes uneven wearing of the feet and, possibly, strain on the joints. The opposite problem is that of toes turning out ('splay-footed'). A splay-footed horse may be prone to brushing and/or dishing.

The hind feet bear less of the stationary horse's bodyweight and are more oval in shape than the forefeet. As with the forefeet the slope of the hoof wall when viewed from the side should be continuous with that of the pastern and, when viewed from the front, the toe should point straight forwards.

Further information on hoof conformation is to be found in another book in this series, *The Horse: The Foot, Shoeing and Lameness*.

AGEING THE HORSE

The gauge used to tell a horse's age is through the stage of development and wear of the teeth. Unfortunately no two horses' mouths are alike, so age assessment can be far from accurate!

Adult geldings normally have forty teeth: twelve incisors, twenty-four molars and four tushes. Mares do not normally have tushes, although it is not unknown for a mare to develop them. Some horses also develop wolf teeth.

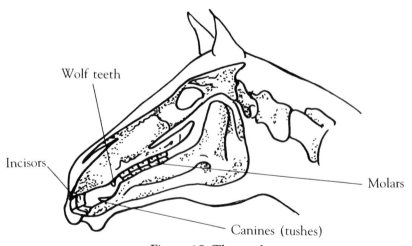

Figure 15 The teeth

The Incisors are biting teeth at the front of the mouth and are referred to as centrals, laterals or corners according to their position.

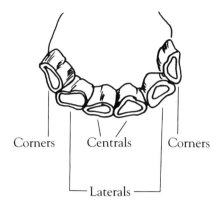

Corners | Centrals | Corners

Laterals

Figure 16 The corner, lateral and central incisors

The Molars are grinding teeth situated at the back of the jaw. These wear with use, resulting in sharp edges. The surfaces or 'tables' wear irregularly, resulting in sharp ridges needed for mastication. However, the grinding action leaves sharp edges on the outer aspects of the upper row and inner aspect of the lower row; these need to be rasped at least once a year.

The Tushes are sometimes known as canine teeth. They appear in geldings when they are about five years old.

Wolf teeth appear in the upper jaw and may interfere with the action of the bit, causing discomfort, in which case they will have to be removed by a vet.

The parts of a tooth are:

Root canal. The hollow root within the jaw.

Pulp cavity. The cavity in the fang containing nerve and blood vessels. (The bulk of the tooth consists of dentine, a mineralized tissue with a composition similar to bone.)

Neck. Point at which the gum and tooth meet.

Crown. Visible part of the tooth.

Enamel. Outer coating of the tooth.

Table. Biting or wearing surface.

Mark (Infundibulum). A blackened depression in the table of the incisors which becomes worn away with the wear of the tooth. Surrounded by a ring of enamel. Sometimes referred to as the 'cup'.

Dental star. Dark line between the mark and the front edge of the tooth. Caused through wear, it is the pulp cavity (fanghole) which now contains dentine coming into appearance.

Galvayne's groove. A dark line which grows downwards from the top of the upper corner incisor, starting when the horse is approximately nine years old.

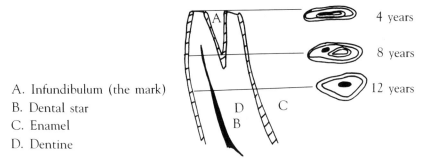

A. Infundibulum (the mark)
B. Dental star
C. Enamel
D. Dentine

4 years
8 years
12 years

Figure 17 Section through tooth

When trying to assess a horse's age, ensure that he wears a headcollar with rope attached, but do not have him tied up. Some horses become upset when having their teeth examined and may pull back suddenly. Without making any quick movements, try to steady the head with one hand over the nasal bones and encourage the horse to open his mouth with the other.

Check both sides of the mouth, as they may differ. As the horse gets older it becomes more difficult to age him accurately. Also, horses who crib-bite wear down the incisors more rapidly, so will have an older looking mouth. Stabled, corn fed horses may wear their teeth down more rapidly than those permanently out at grass.

Table 1. How Teeth Change With Age

Age in Years	Appearance
One	Six neat white incisors (milk teeth) at the top and bottom. The corners do not meet.
Two	Corners only just meet.
Two and a half	The two centrals are replaced by permanent adult teeth and are in wear by three years.
Three and a half	The laterals are replaced by permanent teeth, in wear by four years. The mark extends across the table. Tushes start to emerge in the gelding.
Four and a half	Corners replaced with permanents, in wear by five years. Tushes emerge fully.
Six	All teeth now in wear. Upper corner incisor extends beyond lower corner incisor. Mark ('cup') almost gone from centrals.
Seven	Mark gone from centrals and laterals. Dental star begins to show in centrals. Hook appears on the end of the top corner incisors — the 'seven year hook'.
Eight	Seven year hook worn away. Mark gone from all incisors. Dental star clearly apparent in centrals.
Nine	Dental star appears in lateral incisors. Galvayne's groove appears on the upper corner incisors. This extends downwards over the next ten years.
Ten to Twelve	All incisors have a dental star. The tables now appear round instead of oval. At eleven years there may be a slight hook on the upper corners. From the age of twelve it becomes more difficult to accurately age a horse.
Thirteen to sixteen	The tables now appear triangular. Galvayne's groove extends down the tooth.
Twenty	Galvayne's groove starts to disappear. The teeth start to grow out at an angle. The pulp cavity fills up and the tooth is slowly pushed up, giving the appearance of longer teeth. The gums also recede slightly.

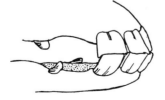

Figure 18 A seven-year-old mouth

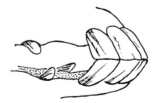

Figure 19 An aged mouth (approximately fifteen years)

THE HORSE IN MOTION

The walk and trot can be assessed both in hand and under saddle. The steps in all gaits should be level and even with no signs of unsoundness. When looking to see if the strides are straight and even, view the horse moving away from and towards you, and from the side.

The walk

There are four steps to the stride. Each step should be of even length and the hoofbeats should be heard with equal intervals between each. There are always two or three feet on the ground at any given time and thus no period of suspension. The walk is a lateral gait, the sequence of footfall being inside hind, inside fore, outside hind, outside fore or, in the same sequence, starting with the outside hind. There are four variations of walk: collected, medium, extended and free.

Qualities of a good walk

Hoofbeats distinct and regular.

Even, unhurried steps. The hind feet should step beyond the prints left by the forefeet, that is, overtracking.

A clear lifting of the feet must be visible as opposed to dragging the feet with little knee or hock action.

The walk must appear purposeful and unconstrained.

The head will nod rhythmically.

The trot

There are two steps to the stride. The horse springs from one diagonal pair of legs to another with a period of suspension in between. There are four variations of trot: collected, working, medium and extended.

Qualities of a good trot

Regular two-time rhythm with even, unhurried strides.

Except in collected trot (see Variations within the gaits) the hindquarters must be engaged enabling the hind foot to, at least, step into the print left by the forefoot, that is, tracking up.

The joints must flex, ensuring that the feet are not dragged.

When moving towards the observer, the trot must appear straight.

When considering the quality of the trot watch for brushing and/or dishing and listen for forging, that is the toe of the hind shoe striking the heel or inner toe edge of the fore shoe.

The canter

There are three steps to the stride, the sequence of footfall being outside hind, inside hind together with outside fore, inside fore, followed by a period of suspension. There are four variations of canter: collected, working, medium and extended.

Qualities of a good canter

Rhythmic three-time beat, not four-time which denotes lack of impulsion or balance.

Strides even, unhurried and balanced, with good cadence.

Hindquarters must be engaged with active hocks.

The canter must be united and straight. (In the disunited canter, the hind foot on the same side as the leading forefoot impacts before the hind foot diagonally opposite the leading forefoot). Hindquarters must not swing in or out.

The head moves rhythmically in relation to the stride cycle. An exaggerated nodding up and down indicates a lack of impulsion and can generally be corrected by increasing the activity of the hindquarters and making the horse go forward more positively.

The gallop

There are four steps to a stride, the sequence of football being (with the left foreleg 'leading'): off hind, near hind, off fore, near fore, followed by a moment of suspension.

Qualities of a good gallop

The four-time beat should be regular and rhythmic.

There should be long, even strides.

The centre of gravity is moved forward and balance maintained.

The horse must remain straight.

Variations within the gaits

As schooling progresses so the basic gaits can be shortened or lengthened and the horse's outline changed accordingly. It is not the purpose of this book to discuss how these variations are achieved, but a brief description of the main principles is given below.

Collected

The steps are uniformly shortened, even and elevated. At walk, the hind feet track up; in trot and canter the hind feet will fall just behind the prints made by the forefeet. The hindquarters are very actively engaged, resulting in a lightening of the forehand. The horse remains on the bit with the front line of the face slightly in front of the vertical.

Working

Formerly described as 'ordinary', working trot and canter represent the movement of a well made but untrained horse, and are used in the earlier stages of training. In terms of stride lengths, the gait falls between collected and medium; the horse should track up and remain on the aids, balanced with active hindquarters.

Medium

The strides are longer than the working variant, but shorter and rounder than the extended. They should be very unconstrained, with plenty of active engagement of the hindquarters. The horse remains on the bit but with the head and neck lower than in working or collected gaits. The front line of the face is a little more in front of the vertical.

Medium walk is the initial walk used for all horses. In both medium trot and walk the hind feet must overtrack.

Extended

The steps are evenly lengthened as much as possible without the horse being hurried into loss of regular rhythm. Therefore, the overtracking is more pronounced than in the medium gaits. As the steps lengthen, so the head and neck lower. The hindquarters are actively engaged producing lively impulsion, but the horse must remain calm and light.

Free gaits

The horse is allowed to relax on a long rein and stretch the head and neck downwards, but he must remain active and straight. The free walk is most normally used as a means of relaxation after a period of hard work.

Faulty action

Conformation defects and faulty joint action may lead to the following faults:

Dishing. The forefeet swing outwards which may exert additional stress on joints, especially on hard ground. This fault is not desirable in a horse required for showing or dressage and may be associated with brushing.

Plaiting. The opposite of dishing, in that the forefeet swing inwards.

Brushing. The insides of the lower limbs 'brush' or knock together, which can cause serious injuries if protective boots are not worn. There are many causes of brushing, including poor conformation and unfitness.

Speedy cutting. High brushing sustained at speed and whilst jumping.

Overreaching. The toe of the hind shoe catches the heel of the forefoot. Serious bruising and other injuries can result.

Forging. The toe of the hind shoe catches the heel of the fore shoe causing a clicking noise. In some instances the fore shoe may be torn off completely.

Daisy cutting. Sweeping steps with insufficient knee action, whereby the feet only just clear the ground.

High knee action. This can lead to concussion-related ailments. Horses with a high knee action tend to take short strides and find lengthening difficult. Likewise, the horse with an exaggerated hock action may find it difficult to engage properly and lengthen the strides taken by the hind legs.

A more detailed description of faulty action and its causes and remedies is given in another book in this series, *The Horse: The Foot, Shoeing and Lameness.*

EXAMINATION TO ASSESS CONFORMATION

When looking at a horse's conformation in an examination, students are sometimes given a brief, for example 'A gentleman client has asked you to look out for a hunter for him to purchase. He is keen to hunt at least once a week, sometimes more'. Further information may be given regarding the client's riding ability and amount of money he wishes to spend. In other cases, students are required simply to talk about the horse's conformation. Points to remember in such circumstances are:

1) Before bringing the horse out of the stable ensure that the yard gate is closed. Put on a bridle and pick out his feet, note whether he is shod and, if so, any uneven wear on the shoes.

2) If the weather is very cold, do not leave the horse standing about without rugs. It is necessary to see him without any rugs to assess his overall appearance and proportion but, once this is done, cover at least half his body with his neatly folded rugs.

3) Before you begin talking about his conformation, look in his mouth and assess his age. As mentioned earlier, the age and stage of training can affect the way a horse looks.

4) When talking about conformation, do not be vague. Do not say things such as 'He's a lovely sort' or 'He has a super face'. Be specific! Describe the horse in a logical and precise way. Proceed as follows:

   a) Assess the overall impression – size, weight and type. Is he a 16.1 hh light, middle or heavyweight? Does he look clean bred, that is Thoroughbred, or he is only a percentage, if any, Thoroughbred? Alternatively, is he a cobby or native type?

   b) Work from the head back towards to hindquarters, pointing out the good qualities as well as any weaknesses. Always back up your statements with reasons as to why a defect *may* lead to a particular problem and what effect it may have on the horse's performance. Conformational defects do not *always* lead to problems. Bear in mind any brief you have been given. For example, the hunter we are looking for needs to have very good, sound limbs but need not have the quality of gaits needed for a pure dressage horse or show hack. For example, a slightly pigeon-toed horse need not be written off immediately.

c) Don't be afraid to move around the horse. View him from both sides, standing well back and from the front and rear.

d) When you have talked about his conformation, you will probably be required to assess his action. Look at him from in front, behind and from the side in walk and trot on an even surface. Look for sound, straight movement. Note any outward or inward swings.

When preparing for this phase of an exam, it is essential to:

1) Look at pictures of proven winners in different spheres; show hacks and hunters, dressage, showjumping, eventing, racing and so on. Notice how they are put together. At shows and events, look at different horses and compare qualities.

2) Practise describing horses in your yard. Look in as many horses' mouths as you can to improve your skill at ageing. Also, study the actions of horses when walking and trotting so you are able to detect faults such as dishing and plaiting.

3) Study the horse market to gauge the level of prices expected for different types. Phone up about a few horses and (tactfully) enquire about the prices if they are not printed in the advertisement.

4

THE NERVOUS AND SENSORY SYSTEMS

The horse's perception of the world around him, his responses and reactions to changes in environment are determined by the efficiency of his systems of information and control. These systems are the nervous system, the sensory systems of sight, smell, hearing, taste and touch and the endocrine system — a system of ductless, hormone-producing glands which control the horse's pattern of behaviour.

THE STRUCTURE OF THE NERVOUS SYSTEM

The nervous system consists of a number of separate but integrated sections which monitor, instigate and co-ordinate the body's many activities. Millions of nerve cells (neurones) transmit messages (impulses). The chief elements of the nervous system are:

1) The central nervous system (CNS), which consists of the brain and spinal cord which are protected by the skull and the spinal column.

2) The peripheral nervous system (PNS), which is connected to the CNS and runs throughout the body.

The central nervous system

It is the general function of the brain to co-ordinate the body's activities. Information sent via the sensory nerves is received by the CNS and the horse reacts accordingly.

The brain is housed within the cranial cavity and is composed of the cerebral hemisphere or fore brain, the mesencephalon or mid-brain and the cerebellum and medulla oblongata – the hind brain. The brain is made up of millions of brain cells or neurons, each consisting of a cell body, axon and one or more highly branched dendrites. These cells consume 20 per cent of all the oxygen extracted from the blood; without oxygen the brain cells become damaged and die. The brain has no capacity for cell regeneration.

The spinal cord is made up of many bundles of nerve fibres carrying messages to and from the brain. The nerve pathways cross, resulting in the left hemisphere of the brain controlling all movement in the righthand side of the body and vice versa.

The brain and spinal cord are encased in tough protective membranes called meninges and are cushioned by cerebrospinal fluid. This fluid also assists in the supply of nutrients and oxygen.

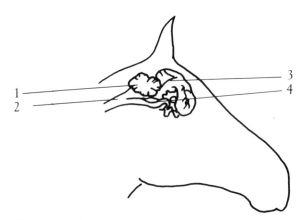

1. Cerebellum (hind brain)
2. Medulla oblongata (hind brain)
3. Cerebral hemisphere (fore brain)
4. Mesencephalon (mid-brain)

Figure 20 The brain

The peripheral nervous system

The peripheral nervous system is divided into two parts: the somatic or voluntary nervous system and the autonomic or involuntary system.

The voluntary system receives information through sensory nerves known as receptors in the musculoskeletal system, eyes, ears, skin, nostrils and taste buds. This information is then taken by the motor nerves to the muscles, thus initiating movement. Motor nerves originate in the CNS.

The involuntary system is concerned with controlling the body's involuntary activities such as the rate of heartbeat, movements of the gut and sweating. This is a very complex system divided into the sympathetic and parasympathetic systems.

The sympathetic nervous system is involved in the fear/fright/flight responses, and the parasympathetic system in vegetative functions such as digestive processes.

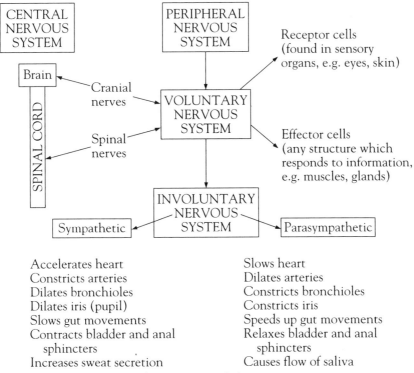

Figure 21 **The structure of the nervous system**

Structure of a nerve cell

The neurons making up the nervous system consist of a cell body containing the cell nucleus and a long tail called the axon. Short branches called dendrites project from the cell body and these conduct messages to the cell body. Contact between the axon of one cell and the body of another is via specialized structures called synapses.

In general, the cell bodies of neurones are located in the central nervous system. The nerves of the peripheral system consist mainly of axons running the whole length of the nerve carrying impulses from the cell body. Cell bodies in the peripheral system, such as sensory and autonomic nerves, collect together in peripheral sites in groups known as ganglia.

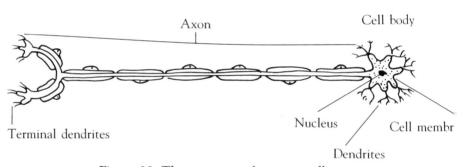

Figure 22 The structure of a nerve cell

Nerve impulses

The way in which a nerve transmits a message is highly complicated and involves the movement of electrically charged particles. The electrochemical messages are able to travel at over 100 metres per second.

While not conducting impulses, the outer membrane of a nerve cell bears a different electrical charge from that inside. Within the cell there is high concentration of potassium and a low concentration of sodium and vice versa on the outer membrane. When a nerve is stimulated, the molecules shift about, allowing potassium ions out and sodium in, which causes an electrical charge to occur. This, in turn, causes charges in the next section of membrane and so the message is passed along the nerve fibre.

The message is passed along the axon in this way and can be transmitted to other nerve cells via the synapses. The electrical impulses do not actually cross these spaces but cause the release of a chemical transmitter substance which makes the following cell develop an impulse. When the impulse reaches the muscle to be moved, the transmitter substance causes changes in the permeability of the muscle fibre membrane, resulting in an alteration in the electrical state across the membrane. This alteration causes the muscle fibre filaments to draw the muscle fibres (myofibrils) along one another, thus resulting in a contracted muscle.

THE SENSORY SYSTEMS

Sight

Because of the positioning of the eyes towards the sides of the head, the horse has wide panoramic vision which is a necessity for survival in the wild. Vision results from the stimulation of light-sensitive cells, causing the creation of a nerve impulse. These impulses are transmitted to the brain for interpretation and 'decoding', thus enabling the horse to perceive his environment.

The structure of the eye

The eyes are set in bony cavities known as the orbits. The eyeball rests on a pad of fat and is held in position by seven muscles, some of which extend down and are arranged around the optic nerve. The protective structures of the eye are:

The eyelids. These are formed by a continuation of the facial skin, covered in short hairs. The upper eyelid is larger and thicker than the lower and is responsible for the opening and closing of the eyes as the lower lid remains fairly still.

The conjunctiva. A thin, moist, transparent membrane which lines the inner surface of each eyelid and extends over the front of the eye. It is very sensitive, being only one cell in thickness, has a low-friction surface to facilitate smooth opening and closing of the eyes and provides protection for the eyeball.

The lachrymal gland. This lies within the orbit above the outer corner of the eye, and continually sheds tears which wash away foreign particles and prevent bacterial proliferation. The tears pass from the lachrymal gland through a pair of lachrymal ducts situated close behind the edge of the eyelids at the inner corner of the eye.

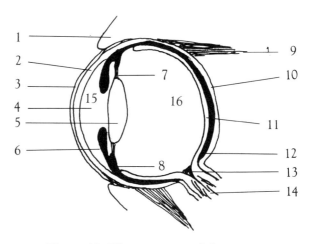

Figure 23 The structure of the eye

1. Upper eyelid
2. Cornea
3. Conjunctiva
4. Pupil
5. Lens
6. Iris
7. Suspensory ligament
8. Cilary muscle
9. Eye muscle
10. Sclera
11. Retina
12. Choroid layer
13. Blind spot
14. Optic nerve
15. Aqueous humour
16. Vitreous humour

Their positioning does not permit certain of the eye structures to be shown on a lateral cross-section. Refer to text for location of the following:

Lachrymal gland
Nasochrymal duct
Tarsal gland
Third eyelid
Corpora nigra

The nasochrymal duct. This lies within the nasal cavity, buried partly in the outer wall of the frontal sinus. Tears originating in the lachrymal ducts drain away down the nasochrymal duct into the nose.

The meibomian or tarsal glands. These are situated along the length of the inner surface of the eyelids and secrete an oily substance onto the edges of the lids to prevent drying.

The third eyelid (membrana nictitans). This membrane lies at the inner edge of the eye and consists of a thin, flexible T-shape of cartilage which is covered in front by the conjunctiva. The stem of the cartilage is embedded in a pad of fat by the side of the eyeball. Pressure on the eyeball causes the fat to push against the cartilage, resulting in the membrane passing over the eyeball. This action removes any foreign particles from the eyeball. Whenever the eye is subjected to pain or threatened from the outside, the eye retracts back into the socket, pressing it against the fat pad, thus causing the third eyelid to cover the eyeball.

The sclera. This is the tough, fibrous white of the eye which forms the outer coating and provides an attachment for the muscles which move the eyeball. It also maintains the shape of the eye and guards the delicate inner layers.

The sight-functional elements of the eye are:

The cornea. This is the front of the sclera. It is oval-shaped in the horse and is transparent to allow the entry of light. This area of the eye is most important for giving a focused image as well as protecting the front of the eye.

The choroid. This is the inner lining of the eye, which has a pigmented muscular continuation called the iris. The choroid layer nourishes the retina.

Aqueous humour. A clear watery fluid which fills the chamber between the cornea and the iris. It maintains the curvature of the cornea and is constantly secreted and drained away.

The iris. This consists of muscle fibres and fibrous tissue interspersed with pigment cells. In an equine eye the pigment is normally very dark. The function of the iris is to regulate the amount of light that reaches the inner part of the eye.

The pupil. This is a circular opening in the iris, the size of which is controlled by the light-sensitive fibres of the iris. In bright light, the pupil becomes narrower and in poor light it becomes dilated.

Corpora nigra. These black, cloud-shaped hanging bodies, sometimes referred to as nigroid bodies, can be seen near the pupil. It is thought that their function is to help regulate the amount of light entering the eye.

The lens. This is an elastic biconcave body which, although transparent, is composed entirely of living cells arranged in layers. It is held in position behind the iris by suspensory ligaments. These connect it to the ciliary body, which consists of smooth muscle. Contraction of the muscle flattens the lens and allows fine focusing of images already roughly focused on the retina by the cornea. In this way, it acts like a camera lens.

Vitreous humour. This clear, jelly-like fluid fills the space at the back of the eye, behind the lens. Its function is to maintain pressure within the eyeball, thus helping to retain its shape.

The optic nerve. Nerve fibres from the retina converge to form the optic nerve. Situated at the back of the eye, this nerve pierces the choroid and sclerotic layers and passes into the brain.

The retina. Situated on the back of the eyeball, this is comprised of approximately ten zones consisting of optic nerve fibres, as well as blood vessels and pigment cells. One of the outermost layers contains light-sensitive photoreceptor cells known as rods and cones.

Rods and cones. These cells receive light, the sensations of which produce nerve impulses which are transmitted via the optic nerve to the brain for interpretation. Rods contain a substance known as rhodopsin or 'the visual purple' and are very sensitive. They are concerned mainly with vision at night or in near darkness. The 'visual purple' is a protein pigment related to carotene which fades after prolonged exposure to very strong light. A good dietary supply of vitamin A (carotene) will help to replenish the 'visual purple' of the rods, so improving night vision. The cones are concerned with detailed vision and colour differentiation under strong light conditions.

Disorders of the eye

BRUISING AND FOREIGN BODIES
Causes
Blow from a projecting branch; hay seed or similar on the eyeball.

Signs
Swollen eyelid and weepy discharge.
Reddened conjunctiva with prominent blood vessels.

Treatment
Bathe with cooled boiled water or eye lotion. Consult the vet if eyeball or lid is damaged or the condition does not improve.

CONJUNCTIVITIS
Causes
Injury, foreign body, allergy or infection, causing inflammation of the conjunctiva.

Signs
The eyelid's inner membrane is inflamed, the eye appears blood-shot with a swollen eyelid and mucosal discharge.

Treatment
Bathe with cooled boiled water or eyewash. Obtain antibiotic opthalmic cream from the vet. If symptoms persist, call the vet. Never use an eye ointment containing corticosteroid if there is any possibility of damage to the cornea, as it can cause ulceration.

CATARACTS

Causes

If congenital, will be present in the foal at birth. It may be progressive, that is to say a small congenital cataract which enlarges throughout the horse's life. The condition may also occur as a result of injury or infection.

Signs

An area of opacity in the lens. The opaque appearance is caused by changes which occur within the layers comprising the lens. Excess fluid between these layers may also account for this appearance. The vet will use an ophthalmoscope to determine the extent of the cataract.

Treatment

The vet will advise.

KERATITIS

Causes

Injury, irritation or infection leading to inflammation of the cornea.

Signs

Watery discharge at first, then the cornea becomes dry. The lids are tightly closed and the horse will show signs of great pain.

Treatment

Call the vet immediately to prevent further deterioration.

ENTROPION

Causes

The eyelid is turned inwards, causing the lashes to irritate the surface of the cornea. This condition affects some newly-born foals.

Signs

Weepy eye and inturned eyelid.

Treatment

Immediately call the vet, who will stitch the eyelid back for a period if necessary. If not treated this irritation will lead to keratitis, ulceration, blindness or complete loss of the eye.

Hearing

The horse has a highly developed sense of hearing; as with the panoramic field of vision, this sense is vital for survival in the wild. In addition to its hearing function, the inner ear is involved with the horse's sense of balance (see *semi-circular canals*, below). As well as performing their sensory roles, the ears also display and express the mood of the horse.

The structure of the ear

The ear consists of three sections:

THE EXTERNAL EAR OR PINNA

The ear is supported by three separate cartilages lying between two layers of skin: the main one is the conchal cartilage, which is capable of depression and elevation, and also sideways, backwards and forwards movement. This enables the horse to direct the ear towards a sound. The inner side of the pinna has a layer of protective hair. The pinna not only protects the middle ear but helps to direct sound into the auditory canal.

THE MIDDLE EAR

This is divided from the external ear by the eardrum or tympanic membrane. Sound is wave-like vibrations of air which vibrate against the eardrum.

Within the middle ear are the three smallest bones in the body, known as the auditory ossicles. These are the malleus or hammer, incus or anvil and the stapes or stirrup. They transmit the vibrations of the eardrum to the oval window, a membrane which closes off the inner ear.

Tubes known as the eustachian tubes connect the middle ear with the back of the throat to help maintain an even pressure on the two sides of the tympanic membrane.

THE INNER EAR

This is tucked into a cavity within the skull for protection. The inner ear houses the cochlea and the semi-circular canals.

The cochlea is a fluid-filled coiled tube resembling a snail shell which receives vibrations passed through the oval window from the stirrup. These vibrations are then converted to nerve impulses which are transmitted to the brain via the auditory nerve and are perceived as sound.

The semi-circular canals are set at right angles to each other in order to monitor angular movement of the head in any direction. They are lined internally with specialized hairs and contain jelly-like fluid which in turn contains minuscule crystals of calcium carbonate, called otoliths. As the head is moved the crystals move and stimulate the hairs, thus triggering off nerve impulses to the brain. (Other vestibules concerned with balance are the ampulla utriculus and sacculus which are interconnected chambers containing hairs, sensory receptors and fluid. Otoliths in this fluid are affected by gravity, causing nerve impulses to be transmitted to the brain.)

1. External ear tube
2. Eardrum
3. Hammer
4. Anvil
5. Stirrup
6. Middle ear (air-filled)
7. Windows
8. Eustachian tube
9. Semi-circular canals
10. Vestibule
11. Cochlea
12. Inner ear (fluid-filled)

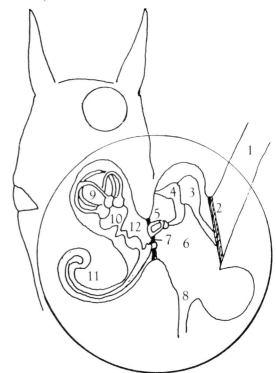

Figure 24 The structure of the ear

Smell

The sense of smell provides horses in the wild with the means of locating edible feedstuffs and fresh water and is, therefore, essential to survival. Stallions are able to detect an 'in-season' mare and horses use their nostrils and sense of smell as a means of getting to know each other — in particular during mare and foal bonding.

The structure of the nose

The nose consists of:

The nostrils. The entrances to the nasal chamber, the rims of which are held open by supporting cartilage. The nostrils are capable of dilation to increase the intake of air and the capacity to smell.

The false nostril. This blind pouch extends back from the nostrils for approximately 10 cm (4 in) and is lined by a continuation of the skin of the face, with some fine hair acting as filters.

The turbinate bones. These lie back within the nasal chamber. They are covered in a mucus-secreting membrane which has many microscopic projections (cilia) growing from it. The olfactory cells, those concerned with smell, are situated in the mucous membrane. These cells are neurones, the cell bodies of which are in the epithelium. A single dendrite extends from the cell body to the free surface, where it branches into fine sensory cilia. Once filtered, warmed and moistened within the nasal chamber, inspired air passes over these sensory cilia. It is thought that molecules of chemical vapour carried in the airstream are deposited on the mucus and stimulate the cilia. These pass the message on to the cell bodies beneath them, initiating a nervous impulse which travels along the fibres from the olfactory cells to the embedded olfactory bulbs which are directly linked to the brain.

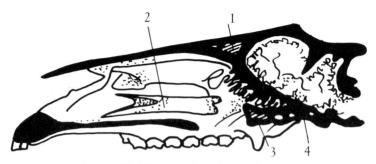

Figure 25 The nasal cavity and sinuses
1. Frontal sinus 2. Turbinate bones 3. Palatine sinus 4. Sphenoid sinus

Taste

The sense of taste is closely associated with that of smell. Horses are suspicious of strange smelling substances and dislike bitter or sour tasting foods. This instinctive reaction affords protection against the ingestion of poisonous substances.

The structure of the mouth

The lips. Covered in feeler hairs, the lips are used to 'sort' through grain and grass while the nose verifies the edible quality of each substance. The lips help to grasp food and stalks, enabling the incisor teeth to bite off the desired fodder.

The taste buds. These cells are found mainly on the tongue and, to a lesser extent, on the palate and in the throat. The taste buds are found in association with thousands of papillae, which form the mucous membrane covering the tongue. Foodstuffs are tasted through being mixed with saliva which dissolves the chemicals within that foodstuff. The dissolved chemicals are spread over the taste buds and passed to the taste receptor cells which are embedded within the papillae. These cells are stimulated and their impulses travel along the nerve fibres to the brain. According to the position of the taste buds, a different nerve transmits these impulses. The brain then sorts out the messages, and identifies the different tastes. Dry feedstuffs have no taste; it is only through being moistened that the receptor cells can be stimulated.

The salivary glands are arranged in pairs and are stimulated by the thought, smell and anticipation of food. They are the parotid glands in the throat area below the ear, the sublingual glands beneath the tongue and the submandibular glands in the lower jaw.

Sensitivity to touch

Sophisticated sensory equipment is located in the horse's skin. Here, various different physical sensations are detected by specialized nerve extremities. These sensory receptors are mechanoreceptors, concerned with touch and pressure and thermoreceptors, concerned with heat and cold. Stimulation of these receptors enables the horse to be aware of his environment; excessive stimulation of any of these receptors causes pain to be felt.

Pain is one of the most important sensations, as it actively helps to keep the horse alive. Horses quickly learn to evaluate the experience of pain and take action to avoid its repetition. It is for this reason that electric strip fencing may be used successfully with many animals. It is often also the reason why some horses go badly for ignorant riders, bucking them off and/ or refusing to jump in order to avoid the pain inflicted upon them by the careless use of rough hands and/or ill-fitting and severe equipment.

Because of the varying number of sensory receptors in each area, some areas of the skin are more sensitive than others. The muzzle is very sensitive because of the long feeler whiskers which pass messages on to the many sensory receptors in the muzzle.

When sensory receptors are stimulated, nerve impulses travel via the spinal cord to a centre in the brain known as the thalamus. This sorts the different impulses into similar groups and passes them on to the sensory cortex, the area of the brain which analyses sensations more finely. Below the thalamus is a smaller structure, the hypothalamus, a nerve control centre which, apart from being concerned with autonomic sensations of hunger and thirst, is responsible for maintaining the body temperature in response to sensations of heat and cold. This region of the hypothalamus can be described as a thermo-regulatory centre, acting rather like a thermostat.

The skin

The skin is the tissue forming the outer covering of the body and is the largest of the body's organs. It is composed of two layers: the underlying dermis, richly supplied with blood vessels and nerve endings, and the tough outer epidermis.

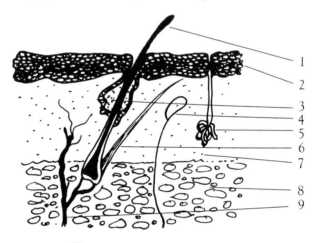

Figure 26 The skin

1. Hair	4. Nerve cell	7. Dermis
2. Epidermis	5. Sweat gland	8. Subcutaneous fat
3. Sebaceous gland	6. Hair erector muscle	9. Blood capillaries

The dermis

This inner layer of the skin contains blood vessels, nerve fibres, lymphatic vessels, heat sensors, glands and hair follicles. The dermis is built around a network of protein fibres which give the skin its elasticity and strength. Healthy skin should feel elastic and supple. The sebaceous glands are closely associated with the hair, secreting an oily discharge known as sebum into the hair follicle. This lubricates the hair and surrounding skin whilst helping to protect against the drying effect of the sun's rays and acting as waterproofing. The sweat glands are little coiled tubes which run through the dermis to emerge on the surface of the epidermis. Through the discharge and evaporation of sweat, the body can be cooled and some waste products, such as urea and lactic acid, excreted.

Lying below the dermis is the subdermal layer, a layer of loose connective tissue between the skin and muscle. Subcutaneous fat stored here provides insulation, cushions muscles and nerves and serves as an energy store.

The epidermis

This is a layered arrangement of cells, of which the top layer is constantly being shed. The lower layers of cells move up to replace those lost and, as they move further away from the source of blood and nutrients in the underlying dermis they degenerate, fill up with granules of the protein keratin and die, forming scurf. This scurf must be regularly cleaned from the surfaces of a working stabled horse to enable the skin to perform its other functions successfully. The sweat and oil glands situated in the dermis pass through the epidermis to the surface, forming openings known as pores.

Vitamin D is synthesised in the epidermis when it is exposed to sunlight.

Hair

The epidermis is covered with hair, which plays an important role in stabilizing body heat. (Some hairs, such as the whiskers on the muzzle, act as a sensory antennae.) Each hair has its own erector muscle which, as a direct response to the skin's sensation of cold, enables it to stand on end. In the winter the horse adapts to the cold weather by growing a thicker, longer coat.

Hair is coloured by its pigment; white hairs have no pigment. Production of pigment, mainly melanin, decreases with age, so as with humans, older horses start to go a little grey. In albinos, the pigment melanin cannot be synthesised because an enzyme is missing as a result of gene mutation and therefore they have white skin and hair. The eyes are more light-sensitive because the iris has no pigment, and they may appear pink.

Modifications of the skin

At the hooves the skin becomes modified; the epidermal cells are filled with hard keratin. At the bodily openings, the skin continues in the form of mucous membranes which are rich in mucus-secreting glands which moisten and protect the delicate surfaces of the nose, mouth, alimentary canal, anal canal and urinogenital organs. These mucous membranes are very well supplied with nerve receptors so are very sensitive to touch and temperature.

Sensory functions of the skin: stabilization of body temperature

In addition to its sensitivity to touch mentioned previously, the skin plays an important role in the stabilization of body temperature. In cold weather, the erector muscle of each hair will contract, causing it to stand upright. Air is trapped between the hairs, helping to insulate the horse. The sebaceous glands become more active, promoting a greasier coat. The blood vessels within the skin constrict, thereby reducing the amount of heat lost through radiation. The horse's metabolic rate (that is, the level at which chemical reactions take place within the cells of the body) also alters in response to extremes of temperature. When the horse is cold the muscles become more toned, gradually becoming tighter and eventually contracting involuntarily, that is, shivering. This produces heat.

When the body becomes heated by muscular activity, hot weather or a combination of both, the superficial blood vessels dilate to radiate more heat, the sweat glands are stimulated to become more active and the metabolic rate decreases. Sweat evaporates off the skin, helping to reduce the body temperature. In humid conditions the sweat will not evaporate easily, possibly resulting in the horse becoming overheated which, in turn, stimulates more sweating. This can lead to the very serious problems of electrolyte depletion and dehydration; great distress is caused to the horse and death may result. In hot, humid countries where horses are expected to compete it is important that facilities for cooling are available and that the body salts lost in sweat are replaced in the form of an electrolyte solution.

The subject of temperature regulation is covered in full detail in another book in the series, *The Horse: Fitness and Competition.*

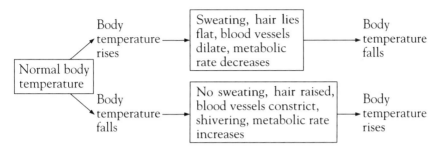

Figure 27 Regulation of body temperature

Non-sensory functions of the skin

The skin also acts in the following ways:

As a barrier. The skin is tough and elastic to help prevent tearing. It acts as a barrier against ultra-violet light, mechanical, thermal and chemical assault. Its relatively impermeable surface prevents excessive dehydration and acts as a barrier to invasion by micro-organisms. After injury to the skin, care must be taken to prevent infection. Subcutaneous fat helps to protect the body against odd knocks. The skin is 'waterproofed' by sebum which, in addition to repelling water externally, also keeps moisture in. The ultra-violet rays of the sun are absorbed by the pigment of the skin, their effect having been weakened by the hair. A grass-kept horse may suffer from a sunburnt nose in sunny weather because of the lack of pigment and hair over the sensitive muzzle area. Greys are especially prone to this painful condition and should be protected by the use of a sunscreen lotion or cream.

As camouflage. In the wild, camouflage is an important survival aid. Moorland ponies are coloured to blend in with the foliage, bracken etc. of their habitat. Another member of the equine family, the zebra, is striped to aid survival in a very different landscape.

As an excretory organ. This is a minor function. Some waste products are excreted in solution with sweat. For this reason, the pores of the working horse must be kept clear through regular grooming. Sweating plays a major role in the cooling process and in this context is also classified as a sensory function. Large amounts of salt are lost through sweating, particularly during strenuous activities. It is important that these salts are replaced to ensure the normal functioning of the body cells.

THE ENDOCRINE SYSTEM

Various bodily functions are controlled by the hormone-producing endocrine glands, which work in collaboration with the nervous system. While the nervous system is concerned with quick or immediate actions, the endocrine system produces various hormones which control processes such as growth, metabolism, conception, gestation, parturition and development. Hormones are organic compounds produced in one part of the body and then transported to another part where they produce a response.

Endocrine means 'internal secretion'; the endocrine glands are ductless and release their hormones directly into the bloodstream. In this respect they differ from the glands of external secretion (exocrine glands), which emit their products to the bodily surfaces and digestive tract via ducts.

The pituitary gland

This small gland is positioned at the base of the brain, to which it is attached by a stalk. It is often referred to as the 'master gland' because of its importance in overall development and the control it has over most of the hormonal system. The pituitary gland has two main lobes, the anterior and posterior, the more important of which is the anterior.

The hormones produced by the anterior lobe of the pituitary are:

Thyroid stimulating hormone (TSH).

Prolactin which influences lactation.

Luteinizing hormone (LH).   ⎱ stimulate secretions of
Follicle stimulating hormone (FSH). ⎰ the ovaries and testes.

Adrenocorticotrophic hormone (ACTH) which controls the adrenal cortex.

Somatotrophin which controls the growth of tissues and influences the metabolism of fats and sugars and is referred to as growth hormone (GH).

Hormones produced by the posterior pituitary gland are:

Vasopressin, which acts upon the kidneys to control the body's water content and is therefore known as antidiuretic hormone (ADH).

Oxytocin, which is mainly involved in labour, helping with the contraction of the uterus, and also assists in the secretion of milk.

The thyroid gland

This gland has two lobes, one being located each side of the larynx. The thyroid produces hormones of two types.

Iodine-containing hormones T3 and T4

T4 is converted to T3 (thyroxin) in general circulation. Secretion of these hormones is regulated by TSH from the anterior pituitary gland. The thyroid gland absorbs materials including iodine from the bloodstream to produce thyroxin. The functions of thyroxin are:

To regulate the metabolic rate.

To maintain levels of heat production.

To influence the absorption of sugars by the intestines.

To influence blood-cholesterol level.

To stimulate energy production in cells.

In youngsters, this hormone works in conjunction with the growth hormone, so is important for growth.

A shortage of iodine will affect the operation of the thyroid gland, resulting in a lower resistance to cold and a lack of energy.

An overactive thyroid increases the metabolic rate, resulting in rapid heartbeat, high blood pressure and weight loss.

Calcitonin

This regulates calcium levels in conjunction with parathyroid hormone. Calcitonin lowers blood calcium by inhibiting decalcification of bone. Secretion of calcitonin is controlled directly by levels of calcium in circulation and is independent of the anterior pituitary gland.

The parathyroids

These are four tiny glands which are attached to the rear surface of the thyroid but actually have little to do with the main gland. Parathyroid hormone (PTH) is vital to the metabolism of calcium and phosphorous. A low blood-calcium level triggers off the secretion of PTH which:

1) Releases calcium from the bones.

2) Acts on the kidneys to reduce calcium excretion and increase phosphate excretion, the effect of which is to boost the level of calcium circulating within the blood.

3) Promotes calcium absorption from the intestine. This effect involves Vitamin D.

When the blood-calcium level is high the sequence is reversed.

Since only small quantities of PTH are produced this results in calcium being laid down in the bones. An in-foal mare must be adequately supplied with calcium to prevent the loss of her own skeletal calcium deposits.

The adrenal glands

One adrenal gland lies on each side of the spinal cord in close proximity to the kidneys. Each gland has two layers, each layer having its own distinct endocrine function.

The outer layer produces steroid hormones known as corticoids.

There are three classes of corticoids:

1) Mineralocorticoids (aldosterone). These are concerned with fluid and electrolyte balance. Their secretion is controlled by renin/angiotensin from the kidneys and their effect is to favour sodium retention in the kidneys.

2) Glucocorticoids. These are concerned with the metabolism of carbohydrates, raising the blood sugar and causing an increase in liver glycogen. Secretion is under the influence of ACTH from the anterior pituitary.

3) Sex hormones. Small amounts are secreted and they supplement the gonadal sex hormone secretion.

The inner layer (medulla) produces adrenalin and noradrenalin. The secretion of the hormones is directly controlled by the sympathetic nervous system. A response to the emotion of fear is known as the 'fright, flight, fight' response. Fear triggers off the following chain of events: the frontal lobe of the brain is stimulated by nervous impulses which lead to the hypothalamus and then directly to the adrenal medulla. The direct nervous control of adrenal medullary secretion permits a rapid response to stressful stimuli. The rapid release of adrenalin causes the pupils and bronchioles to dilate, the heart rate increases and blood pressure increases as blood vessels constrict. The bladder and bowels may evacuate. Horses in a stressful situation will respond to this flight or fight sensation accordingly.

Noradrenalin is a substance chemically identical to adrenalin, but is also a nerve transmitter substance. Noradrenalin is produced at the synapses of nerve cells of the sympathetic nervous system and has the same effect in preparing the horse for 'flight or fight'.

The pancreas

Located behind the stomach, next to the duodenum, the pancreas has both exocrine and endocrine functions as it secretes digestive juices and two hormones. The pancreatic juice is made up of various enzymes and is released into the duodenum via the pancreatic duct.

The endocrine function of the pancreas is of great importance since it is concerned with the maintenance of the blood-glucose level. The glandular tissue of the pancreas is interspersed throughout with small masses of special endocrine cells called islets of Langerhans which produce the hormones glucagon and insulin.

Glucagon encourages the breakdown of glycogen, the carbohydrate stored in the liver, to glucose. Through the utilization of glycogen the blood-glucose level is raised.

Insulin promotes uptake of glucose by most cells, particularly those of the liver, skeletal muscles and adipose tissue (fat). The glucose is then converted to glycogen and fat. Insulin inhibits the further breakdown of glycogen to glucose which has the effect of lowering the level of glucose in the body. In conditions where insulin cannot be produced in sufficient quantities, sugar diabetes results. This is, however, very uncommon in horses.

Release of both hormones is primarily controlled by plasma concentration of glucose. The endocrine functions of the pancreas can be summarized thus:

TOO MUCH GLUCOSE IN BLOODSTREAM (OR PLASMA)

Pancreas secretes less glucagon and more insulin causing the cells to:

1) Increase their uptake of glucose.

2) Convert glucose into glycogen for storage.

3) Convert glucose into fat for storage.

This process decreases the amount of glucose circulating in the body.

TOO LITTLE GLUCOSE IN THE BODY

Pancreas secretes less insulin but more glucagon causing the cells to:

1) Use less glucose for cell respiration.

2) Convert glycogen into glucose for general circulation and use.

This process increases the amount of glucose circulating in the body.

The gonads

These are the sex glands which produce the hormones responsible for giving male and female characteristics.

The ovaries produce oestrogen and progesterone which are essential in the reproductive cycle.

The testes produce testosterone which is responsible for the male characteristics and development.

The sex glands are stimulated by secretions of luteinizing hormone (LH) and follicle stimulating hormone (FSH) from the anterior pituitary gland.

Table 2. A Summary of the Glands, their Hormones and Functions

Gland	Produces	Function
Anterior Pituitary	Thyroid stimulating hormone (TSH)	Stimulates thyroid to produce hormones.
	Prolactin	Influences lactation.
	Luteinizing hormone (LH) Follicle stimulating hormone (FSH)	{ Stimulate secretions of gonads { (sex glands).
	Adrenocorticotrophic hormone (ACTH)	Controls the adrenal cortex.
	Somatotrophin (GH)	Stimulates growth as it controls the growth of tissues, influences the metabolism of sugars and fats.
Posterior Pituitary	Vasopressin (ADH)	Regulates the body's water content through action on the kidneys.
Thyroid	Oxytocin	Active during labour for uterine contractions and production of milk.
Thyroid	Calcitonin	Calcium regulation.
	Thyroxin	Regulates metabolism, stimulates energy production and growth. Influences sugar absorption within the intestines.
Parathy-roids	Parathyroid hormone (PTH)	Vital to the metabolism of calcium and phosphorous.
Adrenal Glands:		
Cortex (Outer Layer)	Glucocorticoids	Steroids involved with metabolism of carbohydrates and proteins.
	Aldosterone	Helps regulate correct water balance.
	Sex hormones	Supplement gonadal sex hormone secretion.
Inner Adrenal Medulla	Adrenalin	Prepares the body for 'flight' or 'fight'.
	Noradrenalin	Assists in the 'flight' or 'fight' sensation.
Pancreas	Glucagon	Facilitates the breakdown of glycogen, thus raising the blood-glucose level.
	Insulin	Encourages the utilization of glucose by the muscles, thus lowering the blood-glucose level.
Gonads: Ovaries	Oestrogen and Progesterone	Essential in the reproductive cycle.
Testes	Testosterone	Responsible for male characteristics and development.

DISORDERS OF THE NERVOUS AND SENSORY SYSTEMS

Impaired nerve supply

Nervous tissue is very susceptible to pressure which, if continual, renders the nerves useless. The nerves will be unable to conduct their messages, leaving the area without sensation. This loss of communication and lack of stimulation means that the muscles supplied by the nerve will waste away, becoming atrophied. Damage to the special nervous tissue of the brain and spinal cord is final as no repair is possible, but damage to peripheral nervous tissue is not always permanent (although regeneration is very slow). Three examples of conditions caused by impaired nerve supply are described below.

Facial paralysis

Causes

The nerves supplying the muscles of the lips, nostrils, cheeks, eyelids and ears pass along each cheek close to the skin. Along the way they fan out to supply the different muscles. Disturbance of the nerve supply may be caused by a severe blow to the cheek, or pressure from tumours, ill-fitting tack (especially headcollar), enlarged glands or inflammatory processes. Prolonged lying on one side may also be a factor.

Signs

Damage to the superficial nerve endings will cause paralysis of the lips and nostrils on the affected side. Breathing may be laboured because the horse will be unable to dilate the nostril. If one side only is affected, the lip will be drawn towards the healthy side as the muscles of the paralysed side will not be able to work in opposition. If both sides are affected, the horse will drool, with both lips hanging loose. In more serious cases the erector muscles of the ear may be affected.

Treatment

Call the vet. Electrical stimulation of the damaged nervous

tissue may be helpful. Feed soft mashes, bearing in mind that the lips will be unable to grasp the food.

Radial paralysis (dropped elbow)

Causes
Pressure on the musculo-spiral (radial) nerve, usually as it passes over the musculo-spiral groove (at lower front aspect) of the humerus. May be as a result of a kick, fall, fracture of the humerus or prolonged lying on one side.

Myositis (muscular inflammation) of the triceps will show a similar motornerve deficit.

Signs
The knee and fetlock on the affected limb are bent, with the elbow dropped and extended. The horse is unable to bear weight or advance the limb.
Skin sensation to the front outside portion of the forearm is lost.

These signs occur because the radial nerve carries the motor supply to the extensors of the forelimb, the lateral flexor of the knee and the sensory supply to the front outer aspect of the forearm — functions which are lost when the nerve becomes paralysed.

Treatment
Consult the vet. Electrical stimulation of the nerve tissue will help prevent atrophy and massage will help improve circulation. It is important to prevent contraction of the flexors of the lower limb.

Wobbler syndrome

Causes
Pressure on the cervical spinal cord from within the canal. Normally affects rapidly growing youngsters four years old and under.

The term wobbler syndrome has been applied to all horses with signs of ataxia (muscle incoordination) and weakness.

The most common cause is cervical vertebral malformation. Other important causes include equine herpes virus and forms of myeloencephalitis.

Signs
Incoordination of the movements, crossing over of the hind limbs and wobbling from side to side. Symptoms worsen if the horse is turned on a small circle.

Treatment
The only cure is to operate and remove the pressure from the spine, but generally this is not performed and euthanasia is carried out.

Grass sickness

Causes
Paralysis of the gut as a result of degeneration of the autonomic nerves which control gut function. The contents of the paralysed gut become hard, dry and impacted. The exact cause is unknown: one theory is that toxins caused by moulds may be involved.

Signs
Acute cases show acute pain, sweating and rolling. The horse may be constipated or pass very hard faecal matter. Less commonly, there may be acute diarrhoea. The stomach becomes distended with fluid which cannot be moved on and gastric contents may reflux out of the nostrils. There may be paralysis of the oesophagus, causing difficulty in swallowing, and foul-smelling breath. Horses may have muscle tremors and areas of patchy sweating.

Chronic grass sickness also occurs, the signs being more subtle − there is severe weight loss and intermittent colic.

Treatment
The mortality rate approaches 100 per cent and no effective treatment is available at present. The horse rarely survives longer than one or two weeks. Research is being carried out to try and find a cure for this fatal condition but currently, once the diagnosis has been made, euthanasia is generally performed.

After death has occurred, the diagnosis is confirmed through microscopic examination of the mesenteric ganglion (the autonomic ganglion controlling the intestines).

Tetanus (lockjaw)

Cause

The bacteria Clostridium tetani is picked up from the soil via an open wound. Clostridium tetani is an anaerobe, which means it thrives only in the absence of oxygen. Once within a wound, especially a deep puncture wound, the bacteria proliferates producing a very potent toxin which is then absorbed in the general circulatory system. From thereon it affects the central nervous system, causing very distressing symptoms. The topic of disease-producing bacteria is dealt with in greater detail further on in this book (Chapter 8).

Signs

Loss of appetite and loss of desire to drink. Gradually worsening stiffness, muscle tremors and reluctance to move. The forelegs may be splayed and the head and neck outstretched with head and tail perhaps raised. Raising the head and tapping the chin causes the third eyelid to pass over the eye. Sudden sound or exposure to light may send the horse into violent spasms. The jaws become clamped. No urine or faeces will be passed. The horse may become recumbent and be unable to rise. Death occurs if the respiratory muscles are affected.

Treatment

Adhere to the rules of sick nursing, keeping the horse in a quiet, darkened stable and follow the vet's advice. This condition is usually fatal although large doses of antibiotics and tetanus antitoxin *may* be effective if administered early enough.

Prevention

Tetanus toxoid is used to immunize horses against tetanus. It is a 'detoxified' toxin and causes an immune response to be built up for protection against the toxin itself. Tetanus vaccination is extremely effective. The recommended regime is two doses four to six weeks apart (usually in conjunction with the 'flu vaccination), then at one year, then every two years. Vaccination more frequently than once a year is not recommended.

Foals may be vaccinated at three months. Before this, protection may be given using the antitoxin, as the immune system is not mature enough to respond to vaccination. Tetanus antitoxin binds to any circulating toxin and neutralizes it. It will protect an unvaccinated animal for approximately three to four weeks, and is used when a horse of uncertain vaccinal status sustains an injury or is at risk from tetanus infection, for example when foaling. It does not, however give long-term protection. The toxoid can be given at the same time, provided different injection sites are used.

Pregnant mares should be vaccinated with tetanus toxoid one month before the anticipated foaling date to ensure that high levels of protective antibodies are passed to the foal via the colostrum.

Sunstroke/Heatstroke

Causes

Prolonged exposure to great heat causes the heat receptor cells to become exhausted and desensitized. Their paralysis causes the body to overheat as its cooling system ceases to work. The overheating leads to heart and lung failure. Muscular activity and deprivation of fluids will contribute to heatstroke, especially if there is high humidity — the most common scenarios are during transit and working in hot, humid conditions.

Signs

The skin may be covered in patches of thick sweat. Breathing will become laboured, with the horse panting. The muscles will quiver. If the condition deteriorates the horse will collapse and have a rapid, weak pulse and high temperature. The eyes will stare, unseeing. The horse may struggle to rise, but will be unable to as the hindquarters become paralysed. Death may follow within six hours.

Treatment

The main priority is to cool the horse as quickly as possible. Keep the horse in the shade and use a hose or ice packs, cold sponging and fanning, especially over the spine, avoiding the loins and croup. Follow the advice of the vet.

This condition is discussed in full in another book in the series, *The Horse: Fitness and Competition*.

Concussion

Causes

A severe blow to the cranium resulting in a shock and possible bruising to the brain tissues. Haemorrhage may occur in bad cases.

Signs

May occur immediately or be delayed. The horse may stumble, fall and be partially or completely unconscious. The muscles will feel relaxed, the pupils may be dilated or asymmetrical, there will be no reflexes and breathing will be laboured.

Treatment

Call the vet. Keep the body warm if the horse is down, but apply ice packs and cold sponges to the head wound. Provide a comfortable bed and a quiet atmosphere. Feed only laxatives and rest according to the vet's advice.

Stringhalt

Causes

Unknown.

Signs

An involuntary, exaggerated overflexion of the hock during movement; the leg is often flexed then slammed to the ground. This jerking action, which may not be present in every step, can affect one or both hocks.

Treatment

The vet may suggest an operation involving cutting the tendon of the lateral digital extensor muscle for severe cases, but normally it is best left. The horse is classified as unsound.

Shivering

Causes
Unknown. Occasionally this condition may show after an illness or fall although there is no proven connection. The likeliest cause is that of pathological changes in the spinal cord.

Signs
Shivering affects the muscles of the hind limb and tail. Affected horses are unable to move backwards when required to do so. The hind limb is suspended and held away from the body. The muscles contract spasmodically, causing a shivering or shaking appearance.

Treatment
No treatment is available. Horses known to shiver may carry on with their hunting/hacking activities but will eventually lose power from the hindquarters.

Stable vices

Windsucking, crib-biting and weaving which can be classified as nervous habits are discussed in another book in the series, The *Horse: General Management*. Horses who have developed these vices are classified as unsound.

5

THE CIRCULATORY SYSTEM

The circulatory system consists of a network of vessels carrying blood pumped by the heart to every part of the body. The blood travels through arteries as it is pumped away from the heart, and through veins on its return journey. The circulating blood transports essential substances:

Oxygen from the lungs to all of the body cells.

Carbon dioxide from body cells to the lungs.

Nutrients and *water* from the gut to the body cells.

Hormones from the endocrine glands to the body cells.

Antibodies (defence force) to sites of injury or infection.

Heat from the centre of the body or working muscles, distributed as required or dissipated.

Waste products from the body cells to the liver and kidneys for detoxification/excretion.

Sixty per cent of the horse's bodyweight (including blood) is water. Blood plays a vital role in regulating the balance of fluids within the body, which is particularly important in the case of a horse sweating heavily. As blood circulates, it gains and loses substances as follows:

Site	Gains	Loses
Lungs	Oxygen	Carbon dioxide
Intestines	Dissolved nutrients	Oxygen
Body tissues	Carbon dioxide, lactic acid	Oxygen
Liver	Urea	Glucose (stored as glycogen)
Endocrine glands	Hormones	Oxygen
Kidneys	Hormones (renin and erythropoietin)	Salts, water, urea

BLOOD

Blood is a complex vital substance, the main components of which are plasma, red and white cells and platelets.

Plasma

Plasma is a straw coloured liquid composed of serum and fibrinogen, in which all of the other components of blood are suspended.

Serum is 90 per cent water and contains dissolved organic substances: amino acids, lipids, glucose, salts and minerals, blood proteins (including antibodies), urea, hormones, enzymes and carbon dioxide.

Fibrinogen is the important blood clotting protein.

In blood samples, plasma is the fluid which can be collected from a sample which has been prevented from clotting, while serum is the fluid left after a sample has clotted.

Red blood cells

The main function of the red blood corpuscles (erythrocytes) is to carry oxygen from the lungs to the tissues. They are in the shape of biconcave discs which have no nucleus. They are constantly being worn out and replaced. Worn cells are destroyed in the liver and spleen and by-products are excreted in the bile.

New cells are produced in the bone marrow. This process of renewal is speeded up as a horse works harder and faster. Red blood corpuscles contain haemoglobin, the pigment which can bind with oxygen and carbon dioxide. Oxygen is carried from the lungs to the bodily tissues as oxyhaemoglobin. Upon reaching needy tissues the oxygen detaches from the haemoglobin and is diffused through the fine capillary walls. Some carbon dioxide is carried away from the tissue as carboxyhaemoglobin; the rest is dissolved in plasma.

White blood cells

The white blood cells, leucocytes, are colourless and transparent. They are larger than red cells but approximately a thousand times less numerous. Their chief function is to defend the body against disease. They can cross the blood vessel walls to accumulate at sites of injury or infection.

There are five types of white blood cells. The first category, known as granulocytes or polymorphs, originate in the red bone marrow and are divided into:

Neutrophils (approx. 60 per cent), which are a defence against acute infection. They engulf invading pathogens, which are then digested by enzymes. Once a neutrophil is full it dies, resulting in the production of pus.

Basophils (less than 2 per cent), which control inflammation by releasing histamine in response to the presence of an antigen.

Eosinophils (less than 3 per cent), which detoxify foreign proteins by producing enzymes which help break them down.

The second category of white blood cells, known as agranulocytes, originate in the lymphatic system and consist of:

Lymphocytes (approx. 40 per cent), which produce antibodies specific to invading pathogens in order to render them harmless.

Monocytes (less than 2 per cent), which are concerned with less acute infection.

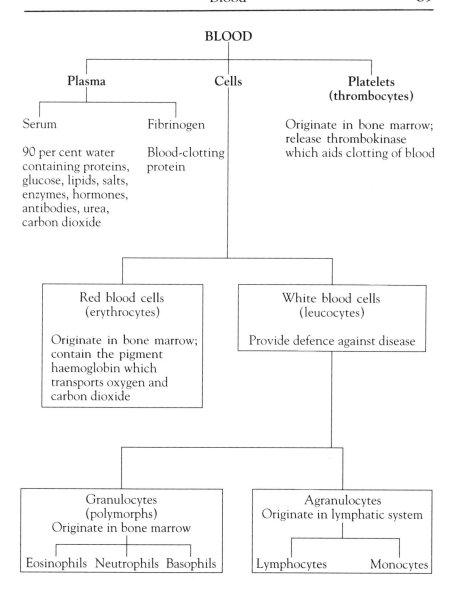

Figure 28 The composition of blood

Platelets

These are the smallest of the blood cells. They originate in the red bone marrow. Platelets release thrombokinase which helps with the process of blood clotting.

BLOOD VESSELS

These are the structures through which blood travels to circulate the body. There are three types of blood vessel; arteries, veins and capillaries. Arteries and veins are mostly named according to the organ that they serve, examples being pulmonary (lungs), renal (kidneys), hepatic (liver) and mesenteric (gut).

The characteristics of the main blood vessels can be summarized thus:

Arteries	Veins
Carry blood away from the heart.	Carry blood to the heart.
Carry oxygenated blood (except pulmonary artery).	Carry deoxygenated blood (except pulmonary vein).
Blood is carried at high pressure.	Blood is carried at low pressure.
Narrow bore highly elastic maintain pressure, widen with heartbeat, giving a pulse.	Wide bore.
Thick, muscular walls.	Thin walls.
No valves.	Valves to prevent backflow.
Branch into arterioles.	Collect from venules.

The capillaries are a network of threadlike vessels extending from arterioles into venules, reaching into every part of the body. Capillaries carrying oxygenated arterial blood converge with those which carry away deoxygenized venous blood. The thin walls of capillaries, one cell in thickness, allow the diffusion of oxygen and dissolved food into the tissues and the removal of carbon dioxide and waste matter. From the capillaries, polymorphs escape to sites of injury to fight infection. The very narrow bore slows the flow of blood between the arteries and veins.

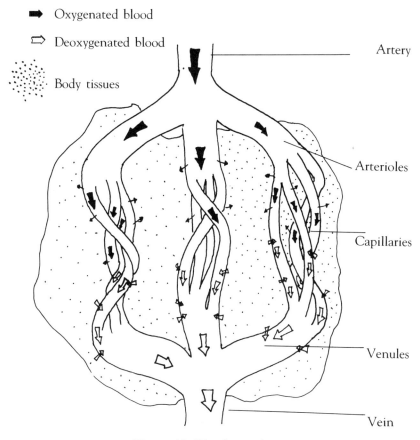

Figure 29 Blood vessels

THE HEART

The heart is situated in the thoracic cavity between the lungs. It is a hollow, muscular organ which can be considered as two pumps working simultaneously. The heart is composed of specialized cardiac muscle which does not fatigue. The average horse of 500 kg (1100 lb) has a heart weighing approximately 4 kg (9 lb).

The heart consists of four chambers; two upper chambers known as atria and two lower chambers known as ventricles. The atria receive blood from the large veins, the ventricles pump the blood out through the large arteries.

The heartbeat

The hearbeat works as follows. Blood enters the left and right atria at the same time. Once full, the atria contract and the valves dividing the atria and ventricles open as the blood is pushed through into the relaxed ventricles. When the ventricles are nearly full the valves close and the ventricles contract, pushing the blood out through the arteries. One-way valves prevent a backflow of blood. The action of heart muscle relaxing before and during the process of filling is known as the diastolic action. The contraction of the heart muscle as it empties is known as the systolic action.

The sound heard when listening to the heartbeat is a very distinct 'lubb-dup'. This can be heard between thirty-six and forty-two times per minute in a healthy adult horse at rest. The 'lubb' sound occurs as the valves between the atria and ventricles close and as the arterial exit valves open, so allowing the blood out to the lungs and body. The harder sounding 'dup' denotes the opening of the valves between the heart chambers and the closing of the arterial valves. The period of silence denotes the heart filling with blood.

THE CIRCULATION OF BLOOD

The heartbeat (assisted, to some extent, by the action of various muscles within the body) powers the two systems of circulation which make up the double circulation of blood within the horse. These are the pulmonary circulation of blood through the lungs and the systemic circulation of blood through the body.

Pulmonary circulation

Deoxygenated blood arrives via the vena cava in the right atrium and then moves down through the tricuspid valve to the right ventricle from where it is pumped through the pulmonary artery into the lungs. Here, carbon dioxide is released through the capillary walls into the lungs, from which it is expelled

→ Oxygenated blood

⇨ Deoxygenated blood

Inhalation — draws oxygen in
Exhalation — breathes carbon dioxide out

Deoxygenated blood is transported to the lungs via the pulmonary artery: carbon dioxide detaches from haemoglobin at the lungs and is exhaled from body

Lungs
Oxygen collected; carbon dioxide deposited

Oxygen attaches to blood pigment, haemoglobin

Pulmonary artery

Deoxygenated blood carries carbon dioxide via the vena cava

Pulmonary vein

Oxygenated blood enters left atrium

Vena cava

Tricuspid valve

Bicuspid valve

Oxygenated blood is pumped out under pressure to the body tissues through the aorta

Body tissues and organs

Aorta

The waste product of tissue respiration, carbon dioxide, attaches to haemoglobin at the tissues

Oxygen deposited at the tissues and used for energy production (tissue respiration): blood is now deoxygenated.

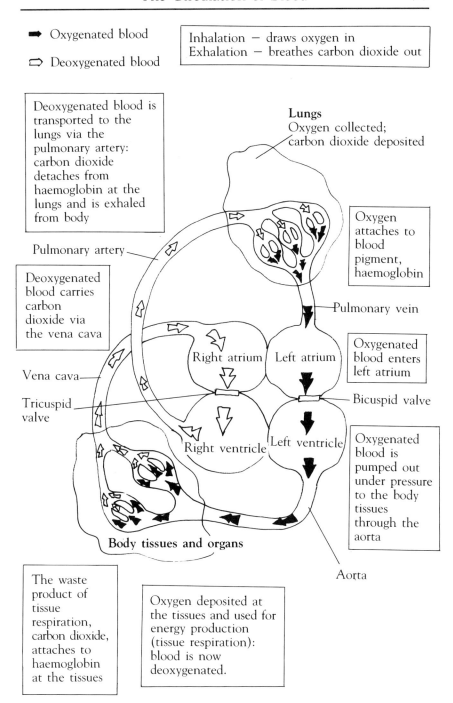

Right atrium | Left atrium
Right ventricle | Left ventricle

Figure 30 Basic pulmonary and systemic circulation

during the process of respiration. Diffusion of oxygen across the thin membranes of the alveoli reoxygenates the blood, which then travels back through the pulmonary vein to the left atrium.

Systemic circulation

Reoxygenated blood moves down through the bicuspid valve from the left atrium to the left ventricle, from where it is pumped out under great pressure through the aorta to the body. Because of the need to send the oxygenated blood out at high pressure, the muscular wall of the left ventricle is thicker and stronger than that of the right ventricle.

The first branches from the coronary arteries supply the heart itself. The many other branches supply every organ of the body, with the first major branch, known as the brachiocephalic, supplying the head and forelegs. The aorta then passes through the diaphragm where a large branch off, the coeliac artery, supplies the stomach, liver and spleen. The mesenteric arteries supply the intestines — the large cranial at the front and the smaller caudal to the rear.

The blood from the intestines is collected in the hepatic portal vein which then subdivides into a capillary network within the liver. The blood is filtered in the liver before going back into general circulation via the hepatic vein which joins the vena cava.

The kidneys are supplied by the renal artery, while the hindquarters are supplied by the iliac arteries. The veins carrying the deoxygenated blood away from the organs and their tissues all converge with the vena cava to enter the heart at the right atrium.

The liver

It is appropriate at this point to include a few important points about the liver, an organ whose functions are so numerous and important that it can be described as the body's metabolic centre. The liver is the largest of the internal organs and has three lobes. It has an excellent blood supply; the hepatic artery

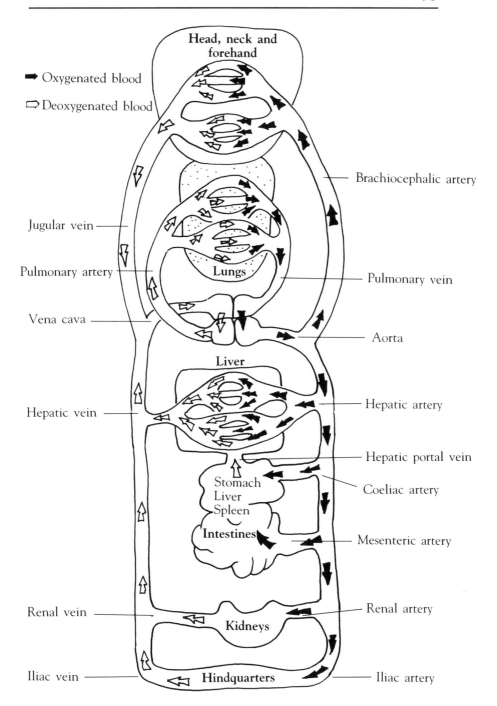

Figure 31 The circulation of blood throughout the body

brings oxygenated blood and the hepatic portal vein brings blood rich in nutrients from the gut.

The liver's many functions include:

1) The breakdown of excess protein, which is then excreted via the kidneys as urea. The excess amino acids are brought to the liver by the hepatic portal vein and are then deaminated by the liver cells, forming ammonia. As ammonia is toxic, it is acted upon by specific enzymes in the liver to form a less toxic nitrogenous compound, urea.

2) Detoxifying waste products and pathogens. In addition to their work on ammonia, the liver cells detoxify many other harmful substances including drugs by absorbing them and changing them chemically.

3) The removal and breakdown of old red blood cells (performed both alone and in conjunction with the spleen). Haemoglobin is broken down by the liver cells and is excreted in the bile, hence the dark colouration of faecal matter.

4) Regulation of body temperature. The liver is an important source of body heat because it has a continually high metabolic rate and excellent blood supply. These factors, coupled with its large size, make it an ideal organ for the steady production and dissemination of heat.

5) The production of bile salts. The liver cells synthesise bile, which flows into the duodenum and emulsifies lipids.

6) The production of cholesterol and maintenance of lipid levels. Cholesterol is a lipid-like substance; the precursor for certain digestive acids and steroid hormones. The liver cells remove lipids from the blood and either break them down or alter them for storage as body fat.

7) Maintenance of blood-glucose levels. As a result of the actions of the two hormones, insulin and glucagon, glucose is either utilized or stored in the liver to regulate the amount in circulation.

8) Storage of iron and vitamins A, D and B12.

9) Synthesis of blood plasma proteins such as fibrinogen, albumen and globulin.

10) Storage of blood. The large veins in the li... serve as a blood reservoir. Together with the regulate the amount of blood in general cir...

FITNESS AND THE CIRCULATORY SYSTEM

Training and fitness work have a very noticeable effect upon the circulatory system. As the duration and level of exercise increase the muscles contract more often, resulting in the need for more oxygen and the removal of more waste products.

In order to cope with these extra demands the circulatory system has to work efficiently. With work, the heart becomes increasingly efficient as it pumps more blood around the body with each cardiac cycle. It also increases in size.

As a response to the increase in demand for oxygen and removal of waste products, more capillaries are formed, so giving a greater surface area for the process of gaseous exchange. In an unfit horse these adaptations are reversed. A fit horse will:

1) Have a slower resting heart rate (may be as low as twenty-six beats per minute).

2) Show a less marked increase in heart and respiratory rates after strenuous exercise.

3) Recover after exercise more quickly, that is, the respiratory and heart rates return to normal more quickly. (When the horse gallops, his heart rate may reach a maximum of 260 beats per minute).

During strenuous exercise, especially in an unfit horse, it is difficult for the body to provide enough oxygen for the muscle cells to cope with the workload. The muscles are forced to work anaerobically, resulting in lactic acid production. When lactic acid accumulates in the muscles, muscular fatigue and pain result. The oxygen debt is 'paid off' after the exercise and it is this which causes the respiratory rate to continue to be elevated when the horse is 'cooling off'. This process of anaerobic respiration is discussed in another book in this series, *The Horse: Fitness and Competition*.

Methods of monitoring heart rate

The horse's heart rate can be monitored by the following methods:

Taking the pulse. This is done at a point where an artery passes over bone, close to the surface of the skin. The pulse may be felt in the facial artery on the inner edge of the lower jaw-bone, or on the inside of the foreleg, level with the elbow, in the radial artery.

Stethoscope. This is placed just behind the horse's left elbow. The stethoscope may be used by the rider/trainer and is particularly useful when monitoring fitness.

Pulse monitor. Electrodes pressed onto the horse's skin record the heart rate, which can be read instantly by the rider on a digital display which is normally strapped to the wrist. These monitors are very useful when gauging the progress of fitness in the interval training programme.

Electrocardiogram (ECG). Specialized equipment used by the vet can measure and record the level of electrical activity created by the nervous impulses in the heart.

When cardiac muscle is relaxed it has a negative electrical charge. In this state, it is said to be polarized. A flow of positive charges into the muscle cells cause them to become positively charged — depolarized. When cardiac muscle cells are depolarized they contract. The contractions are shown on the ECG trace as waves. These waves are identified as P, Q, R, S and T waves. The P wave results from atrial depolarization and the QRS complex from ventricular depolarization. The final T wave represents ventricular repolarization (see Figure 32).

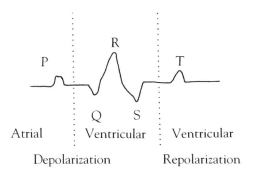

Figure 32 An electrocardiogram trace

The size of the heart can also be gauged as the larger the heart, the longer it will take to contract.

Blood and serum analysis

The various cells are present in the blood in characteristic proportions and analysis of these proportions helps to assess the state of a horse's health. To be of real benefit, tests must be taken regularly so that the individual's normal proportions are known. The correct functioning of the organs and level of fitness of the horse may be tested through the analysis of blood and serum samples in the laboratory. This is a very specialist occupation undertaken by haematologists and biochemists. The results of their findings are then interpreted by the veterinary surgeon.

In order to obtain a true reading, blood tests must be taken before exercise and when the horse is calm. This is because the spleen acts as a reservoir of blood, releasing this surplus whenever the system is under stress, for example, during exercise.

After swabbing the hair with surgical spirit, the vet will insert a needle into the jugular vein and remove approximately 3 ml of blood, which is then mixed with an anticoagulant to prevent it from clotting. A further 6 ml (approx.) is taken and allowed to clot for serum examination. All blood must get to the laboratory within twenty-four hours as it starts to degenerate if kept too long. The absolute number of red and white cells can be determined by manual or sophisticated electronic means.

The different types and proportions of white cells are determined manually by a smear preparation of blood, or by electronic scanning.

The remaining unclotted blood is placed in a tube and spun at very high speeds (centrifuged), causing the cells to fall to the bottom of the tube. Analysis is then made using the following red cell parameters:

RBC. Red cell count — the actual number of red cells per ml of blood.

PCV. Packed cell volume. The proportion of blood cells to plasma is measured as a percentage — this measurement is known as the packed cell volume (PCV). The normal range of PCV is between 34 and 44 per cent. A high percentage PCV can indicate that the horse is suffering from dehydration and/or shock.

Hb. Concentration of haemoglobin g/per ml blood.

McV. Mean (average) red cell volume.

McHc. Mean (average) red cell haemoglobin concentration.

McH. Mean (average) red cell haemoglobin content.

The fluid left after the blood has coagulated is serum — plasma minus the clotting agents. Serum is examined for enzymes, the biological catalysts which cause metabolic processes to occur and for proteins, albumin and globulins.

The veterinary surgeon will take into account the findings of the blood and serum analysis and make his diagnosis accordingly. Conditions commonly diagnosed by these means include:

Anaemia. Indicated by an abnormally low red blood cell count/concentration of haemoglobin.

Azoturia. The severity of azoturia may be gauged by the levels of the enzymes creatine phosphokinase (CPK) and aspartate aminotransferase (AST) found in the muscles. Damage to muscle causes an increase in CPK and AST levels.

Bacterial infection. The total number of white blood cells increases, as does the percentage of neutrophils.

Dehydration. A lack of body fluid causes the PCV percentage to become higher.

Fitness level. A fit horse will have a high number of red blood cells and higher haemoglobin concentration.

Kidney function. Increased quantities of creatine and urea may indicate abnormal kidney function as the kidneys normally excrete them.

Liver damage. Since liver cell damage releases specific enzymes into the circulatory system, raised levels of these enzymes indicate liver damage.

Muscle damage. As mentioned in azoturia, this causes a higher level of CPK.

Parasitic damage. This is indicated by an increased quantity of beta globulin, and a reduction of the blood protein albumin. Migrating worms damage the intestines and blood vessels, causing leakage and loss of albumin.

Viral infection. Typically, in acute viral disease, a reduction in the total number of white cells and reduced number of neutrophils in comparison to lymphocytes is seen — the normal ratio of 60:40 (N:L) becomes 40:60.

In the latter or recovery stages an increase in total white cell count may be seen — this may be caused by bacterial secondary infection.

DIRECT DISORDERS OF THE CIRCULATORY SYSTEM

These are disorders which originate within the system itself.

Anaemia

Signs
External signs:

Poor coat, generally dull and depressed condition.
Pale mucous membranes.
Weakness and lack of appetite.
Reduced stamina and performance.
Increased heart rate − the pulse will be faster as the heart works harder in order to pump any given amount of oxygen around the body.

Blood test will show:

Reduced red blood cell count.
Low haemoglobin concentration.

Causes
The shortage of red blood cells may be caused by:

1) Severe bleeding from a serious wound, serious attack of epistaxis (nosebleed) or other cause such as haemorrhage resulting from ingestion of an anticoagulant such as Warfarin.

2) Actual destruction of red blood cells (haemolytic anaemia). This may occur as a result of viral or bacterial infection, poisoning or a malfunction of the immune system.

3) Dietary deficiency. Poor quality food, in particular folic acid deficiency, affects the output of red blood cells and haemoglobin from the bone marrow.

4) Redworm (Strongylus vulgaris) infestation.

Treatment
Remove the initial cause as appropriate, for example:

Stop any bleeding/treat nosebleeds.
Call the vet to deal with any infection.
Rectify diet − ensure adequate green feed such as grass.
Administer anthelmintics (wormers).
Rest the horse while he regains strength.

Add a dietary supplement to the feed which contains iron, copper, folic acid, vitamin B12 and vitamin E. This is useful for the stabled horse who is unable to take in his own folic acid through grass. There are many specially formulated supplements available to treat and prevent anaemia. The vet may give an injection of vitamin B12 to boost production of haemoglobin.

Prevention
Keep to a well balanced diet using only good quality feedstuffs.
Worm regularly.
Grow herbs in the paddock and feed cut comfrey.
Add a vitamin and mineral supplement to feed.

Shock

Often neglected when discussing disorders of the circulatory system, shock is one of the most important as it is potentially life-threatening. The condition can be defined as a state of progressive circulatory failure in which the primary problem is poor capillary perfusion. The blood pressure may drop, or may remain normal. The output of the heart is insufficient to meet the tissue requirements for nutrition, oxygenation or waste disposal and there is a reduction in the volume of blood circulating within the body. This may be a loss of whole blood, or loss of a fluid component of blood. Examples of the latter would include dehydration, pooling within the intestines, or a mis-match between the circulating volume and the vascular space — that is, when the blood pressure drops.

Signs
The external signs include:
    Apathy and weakness.
    Weak, rapid and irregular pulse.
    Cold, shivering with a 'clammy' feel to the skin.
    Rapid and shallow respirations.
    Temperature below normal.
    Dilated pupils and glazed cornea.
    Darkening of mucous membranes (cyanosis).

These signs are caused by the following physiological changes:
Reduced venous and arterial blood pressure.
Pooling of blood within body cavities or organs.
Lack of circulation (stasis) within capillary network, causing
oxygen starvation.
Increased heart rate to try and meet oxygenation requirements.

Causes
The major causes of such changes, together with their treatments, are listed below.

HAEMORRHAGE
Profuse loss of blood, either externally or internally, will cause
a reduction in the volume of circulating blood. Internal
bleeding may lead to pooling of blood in the body cavities or
organs, so removing it from the circulatory system.

BURNS AND TRAUMATIC INJURY
Tissue fluids accumulate at the site of burns and injury. If the
damage is extensive, proteins leak from damaged capillaries and
large quantities of fluids will be removed from the circulatory
system, causing a reduction in plasma volume, cardiac output
and blood pressure.

Treatment
(Obviously, the vet must be called immediately after an accident
causing either of these conditions. Before he arrives, do what
you can to lessen the degree of shock, for example, stem any
serious bleeding and prevent heat loss — keep the horse warm,
but not too warm. If he is too warm the blood vessels will
dilate, causing a further pooling of blood in the capillaries and
reducing the blood pressure.)

1) Restoration of circulatory blood volume. This needs to be
   done as quickly as possible. Whole blood, plasma or a
   plasma substitute is given by intravenous drip.

2) Administration of oxygen. If the shock is severe enough to
   cause cyanosis (blueing of the mucous membranes caused by
   lack of oxygen to the tissues), then increasing the level of

inspired oxygen will help reoxygenate the blood. A small portable oxygen supply kit is now available for horses.

3) Antibiotics to treat or prevent infection.

COLIC

Any interference with the progress of the intestinal contents constitutes an obstruction. If an obstruction is not diagnosed and treated quickly it can lead to shock. There are two main types of obstruction; − simple, whereby there is no compromise to the blood supply and strangulating, whereby the blood supply is obstructed. If there is interference to the blood supply the risk of death becomes much greater.

Simple obstruction. An example of this would be large colon impaction (constipation). The muscular waves of the intestines increase initially, becoming spasmodic and adding to the discomfort already felt. Large quantities of fluids; saliva, gastric, pancreatic and biliary secretions, accumulate in the upper digestive tract, unable to pass the obstruction to reach the lower, absorbent surfaces. As the intestine becomes distended, more fluid is drawn in from the circulatory system and, as pressure builds up, pain increases. These secretions may remain within the tract, unable to be reabsorbed into the system, or they may be expelled nasally. Body salts and electrolytes are also lost in the fluid. This loss of body fluids from the system causes a reduction in cardiac output and central venous pressure; the horse will then be in a state of shock.

Strangulating obstruction. The blood supply may be obstructed as a result of one of the following:

1) Bowel malposition. Part of the intestinal tract may become trapped in an abnormal position.

2) Twisted gut. The intestinal tract may have twisted over on itself. This is the most serious form of obstruction as blood supply to the twisted portion is immediately lost.

3) Intussusception. A length of the intestine may pass into the length lying just beyond it, rather like a telescope closing up.

4) Hernia (umbilical or inguinal). A loop of gut passes into the hernia sac and becomes trapped as a result of swelling and engorgement of the gut wall. The lack of blood, and therefore of oxygen, to the gut wall causes degeneration of the tissue and allows leakage of bacterial toxins into the abdominal cavity. The toxins are absorbed through the lining of the cavity (peritoneum) into the bloodstream, causing the first stages of endotoxic (septic) shock.

Initially, in cases of strangulating obstruction, the blood vessels dilate and the heart rate increases. As a result of dilation of the blood vessels, the blood pressure drops and the venous return of blood to the heart becomes diminished. The severe drop in blood pressure stimulates the secretion of vasoactive chemicals which cause the blood vessels to constrict. The constriction of the arterioles and venules leads to a further reduced blood flow, resulting in the pooling of blood in the body tissue. Any leaking toxins have a direct effect on the walls of small blood vessels, allowing the escape of blood proteins. This further reduces blood pressure as fluid escapes and pools in the tissues. Pooling results in oxygen starvation within the tissues, causing the cells to switch to anaerobic metabolism. This leads to a great disruption of the pH levels in the cells with a very marked build-up of lactic acid. Death follows within a few hours.

Because of the potential gravity of the condition, as soon as any form of colic is suspected, the vet must be called. Whilst waiting for the vet, walk a colicky horse around to prevent rolling, although if the horse is in pain, reluctant to walk and not trying to roll, there is no need to *force* him to walk.

The vet will assess the condition and treatment will obviously be dependent upon its nature. Early treatments may include painkillers to ease discomfort of an injured horse and anti-spasmodics to ease the passage of an impaction in the gut. Laxatives such as liquid paraffin may be given for impactive colics. An obstruction will require immediate treatment and possibly, depending upon its severity, surgery. Surgery must be carried out within a few hours of a strangulating obstruction occurring.

When nursing a horse who has suffered from shock, keep him quiet and comfortable in a well bedded, airy stable. Follow the appropriate rules of sick nursing and always follow the vet's advice. If in any doubt, write down all information given.

Heart murmurs

Heart murmurs will be detected by the vet during routine examination. Under normal circumstances a smooth, stream-lined flow of blood through smooth, unobstructed vessels is silent. A murmur will be heard in what would normally be a silent period in the cardiac cycle, if the blood is flowing turbulently. Turbulent blood flow results from factors which give rise to changes in velocity, density and viscosity. A common cause is obstruction to the free flow, for example narrowing of the blood vessels or irregularities in the normally smooth edges of the valvular openings. The vibrations of damaged valve tissue may be heard and are known as regurgitation murmurs. Turbulent blood flow through the heart itself may arise as a result of:

Narrowing of the valve opening as a result of heart disease.

Regurgitation of blood through a faulty valve.

Inflammation of the tissues lining the heart — endocarditis.

Compression of vessels by tumours or abscesses.

Having detected a murmur, the vet will consider several factors to determine its significance, because not all murmurs prove to be problematical. These factors include:

Character. The combination of sounds, which cannot be too precisely defined. Generally speaking, the greater the pressure of blood through a small opening, the harsher the sound. A more gentle sound may be heard when there is less pressure, for example stenosis (narrowing) of an atrioventricular valve.

Location in the cardiac cycle. The vet will try to determine whether the murmur occurs during the systolic or diastolic action of the heart, that is during the period of contraction and emptying of a chamber or dilation and filling of a chamber.

The effect of exercise on the murmur. The increased blood flow produced by exercise will often accentuate a murmur. However, some murmurs actually diminish or disappear with exercise and are thought to be insignificant.

Arrhythmia

Arrhythmia may be described as an abnormal and irregular heartbeat caused by a disturbance in the transmission of normal nerve impulses in the cardiac muscle tissue. There are different types of arrhythmia, the most common of which is atrioventricular block. A first-degree block shows on an electrocardiogram as a prolonged (more than 0.4 sec) gap between the P-wave and the QRS complex. A second-degree block shows as the atrial P-wave not being regularly followed by a QRS complex (see Figure 32). It is a normal finding in a fit horse at rest, where the heart rate is low, and it disappears with exercise.

The most common pathological arrhythmia is atrial fibrillation. This is a specific condition denoted by rapid, uncoordinated contractions of the muscle fibres of the atria. The ventricles contract normally but with an erratic rhythm and lowered cardiac output.

The initial signs include a marked reduction in stamina and performance and an irregular pulse. The causes of this condition are not fully understood. The vet may or may not suggest specific treatment, but it may well be necessary to move the horse into lighter work.

Thrombosis

A thrombus or embolism is a blood clot which forms either in a blood vessel or in the heart itself. If the thrombus travels through the circulatory system it may come to rest, causing an obstruction to the blood supply in that area. This is known as thrombosis. The most common sites of occurrence are the points at which the mesenteric artery supplying the gut, and the iliac artery supplying the hindquarters, branch off from the aorta.

Signs

These are dependent upon the site of the blockage. If it occurs in the iliac artery supplying the hindquarters, there will be a degree of hind leg lameness with cramp-like pain. If the thrombosis is within the blood vessels supplying the gut, colic will result.

Causes

The clot may form as a result of larval worm damage within the arterial system. Further damage may occur causing arteritis — inflammation and thickening of the artery walls. If the walls of the arteries become weakened and thinner, an outward bulge may occur, followed by collapse. This is known as an aneurism.

Treatment

Call the vet, who will determine the severity of the condition and treat the colic (if applicable).

If there is any evidence of worm infestation or damage, the horse must be treated with an anthelmintic which is effective against migrating larvae, especially those of Strongylus vulgaris (redworm) which specifically migrate through the cranial mesenteric artery, causing aneurismal damage. Ivermectin is such a drug.

It is essential to maintain a regular worming programme, and this must include unridden youngstock. Although it is possible to treat an existing worm burden in a horse being brought into work, it is not possible to repair damage which has already been caused.

METABOLIC DISORDERS LEADING TO VASCULAR DISTURBANCES

When discussing disorders of the circulatory system it must be understood that, in some instances, the primary cause is not a direct malfunction of this system but the result of a metabolic imbalance. For some conditions, for example laminitis and azoturia, the exact cause is not known and extensive research is still being carried out in order to determine a more exact primary cause.

Azoturia

Also known as: tying-up syndrome, setfast, Monday morning disease, paralytic myoglobinuria, blackwater, exertional rhabdo-myelitis.

Signs

This condition normally affects the fit, stabled horse upon return to work after a period of enforced rest. The horse works normally at first but, a short while later, shows reluctance to move forwards. In mild cases, the muscles of the hindquarters become stiff and tense but improve with gentle walking. This is frequently known as 'tying-up'.

If the horse starts to stagger, sweat profusely and show signs of quickened breathing, the condition is more serious. In very severe cases, the hindquarters are so painful and tense that the horse cannot stand.

Any urine passed will be a much darker colour than normal (reddish brown to almost black) and will have a strange smell. This is caused by muscle fibres being destroyed by the acidic levels thus releasing the pigment myoglobin. Myoglobin is then excreted in the urine.

Causes

Anything which causes an imbalance in the metabolism of carbohydrates may lead to azoturia. This may include:

1) A deficiency in, or imbalance of, vitamin E, selenium, salts and electrolytes.

2) Enforced box rest on normal working rations, particularly if these rations are rich in carbohydrate.

3) Irregular exercise of a fit horse.

4) Excessive exercise of an unfit horse resulting in anaerobic respiration. Lactic acid, a by-product of anaerobic respiration, is carried away in the bloodstream with other waste products. If the lactic acid is not removed quickly enough it builds up in the muscle tissue, causing it to become acidotic. This interferes with normal cell function, resulting in the cramp-like symptoms of azoturia.

Treatment

Immediate action whilst out on exercise is to dismount, slacken the girth and cover the hindquarters with jacket or rug. Then call for assistance and box home.

If the condition is very severe call the vet, who will advise on transporting the horse home — some surgeries have a horse ambulance or specially converted trailer. A horse who cannot stand is obviously in need of specialist equipment to facilitate transportation. Keep the horse as warm as possible while waiting for transport to be organized.

Once home, if you have not already done so, call the vet. Place warm blankets over the quarters to help to relax the muscles. If they are installed, infra-red lamps provide a soothing warmth. (These must be securely installed with all wires safely encased.) Ensure that the horse cannot touch the lamps and that no bedding or clothing can come into contact with them.

Feed very small quantities of hay and laxative bran mashes. (Limestone flour should be added to ensure correct calcium: phosphorous ratio.)

The vet may give anti-inflammatory and painkilling agents such as phenylbutazone. The dark colour in the urine is, as mentioned, myoglobin released from the damaged muscle cells. A build-up of this pigment can damage the kidneys so, in severe cases, fluids may have to be administered to flush the pigment from the kidneys.

Blood testing for levels of enzymes CPK and AST will help to determine the severity of an attack. Rest is essential — the length of the rest period will depend upon the severity of the attack; at all times the vet's advice should be followed. If the horse is worked too soon, further muscle damage may occur.

Prevention

A horse known to have suffered will always be prone to further attacks, so prevention is of great importance:

1) Feed according to the work done. Some of the energy may be provided in the form of fats rather than carbohydrates.

2) Always feed a well balanced diet. Reduce carbohydrates whenever possible and ensure a balance of electrolytes, vitamin E and selenium.

3) Keep feed ahead of work — cut back onto a low carbohydrate diet the day before a rest day.

4) Follow a careful fitness programme so the horse's muscles are never overstressed and follow a regular pattern of exercise.

5) At the start of a schooling session, warm up slowly and thoroughly; at the end of a schooling session, warm down at walk to allow waste products to be removed by the circulatory system.

6) On rest days a horse prone to this condition should not stand in his stable; either lead out in hand or turn out for a few hours.

Laminitis

Laminitis occurs as a result of several physiological changes which take place throughout the body, all culminating in a reduced blood flow through the sensitive laminae of the hoof wall.

Laminitis can affect both horses and ponies, but more commonly affects the latter. Research continues in an effort to determine why some animals are more prone to the condition than others, and what exactly causes it.

Signs

Laminitis may affect any combination of fore or hind feet but, usually, both forefeet are involved. Often, but not always, the feet feel hot, particularly around the area of the coronet. The animal is normally reluctant to move, finding turning particularly difficult. He may shift his weight from foot to foot and will resist attempts to have a foot lifted. The weight is borne on the heels, with the hind feet well under the body and the forelegs extending forward. In severe cases, the horse may sweat and his breathing quicken. He may lie down and be reluctant to stand. There may be a rise in temperature which might go as high as 106 °F (41 °C). The pulse rate may increase to between 80 and 120 per minute: the condition is extremely painful.

The blood pressure rises, causing changes in the blood flow to the feet. This is not yet fully understood as, although the increase in blood pressure causes increased blood flow to the feet the blood flow through the sensitive laminae is decreased. It is thought that blood is 'shunted' from arterioles to venules without passing through the capillary bed of the laminae. There is a strong, bounding pulse in the digital arteries, level with the fetlock, partially the result of pain and the effect of the arterial blood reaching the obstructed vessels within the foot.

The capillary network within the sensitive laminae becomes congested with blood, the pooling of which results in the inefficient exchange of gases, leading to oxygen starvation in the tissue cells of the sensitive laminae. This deprivation causes damage to the tissue, the severity of which is dependent upon the duration of the disrupted blood flow. The damaged tissue swells, forcing the laminae away from the pedal bone. The weight of the horse bearing down on the pedal bone causes further separation. In severe cases the pedal bone may rotate downward and press on the toe area of the sole. This pressure may eventually lead to the death of the tissue in the area (necrosis) which, if not corrected, may lead to the pedal bone penetrating the sole. If this occurs, the prognosis is extremely poor and euthanasia should be considered. Any damage to the tissue of the sole may then lead to secondary infection of the sensitive laminae ('seedy toe'). The rotation of the pedal bone may lead to a convex appearance of the sole and severe lameness.

Causes

As mentioned above, the exact causes are not fully known. However, Laminitis may be divided into two categories:

Traumatic laminitis in which the physiological changes are not the primary cause. For example, concussion may cause bruising and damage to the tissue of the sensitive laminae.

Systemic laminitis which is caused through a culmination of physiological changes in the body.

There are many different factors which, in any combination, may cause a reduction in blood flow through the vessels of the sensitive laminae, and trigger off systemic laminitis. Although horses can be sufferers, it has always been recognized that the 'fat pony on lush grass' is the most likely potential laminitis victim; physiological changes occur as a result of an imbalance in the metabolism. The factors which may bring about these physiological changes include:

1) The production of endotoxins. This may occur in several ways:

   (i) These toxins may be produced within the body as a result of a bacterial infection, for example after foaling there may be retention of the afterbirth leading to infection of the womb (endometritis).

   (ii) As a result of colic — endotoxins released from compromised gut in a strangulating lesion.

   (iii) Carbohydrate overload (from corn or spring grass). This alters the balance of bacteria within the caecum, resulting in production of lactic acid. The change in pH kills some of the Gram-negative bacteria with the resultant release of endotoxins. These are absorbed into the bloodstream, resulting in laminitis.

   (iv) In liver disease. If, for some reason, the liver is damaged and not functioning properly, endotoxins may build up in the circulation, causing laminitis. A blood test would show raised liver enzymes.

2) An imbalance of calcium to phosphorous and of sodium to potassium. These imbalances are thought to affect the passage of electrochemical nerve impulses which could cause paralysis of the muscles of the arterial walls — this would exacerbate the problem of increased blood pressure. Moreover, the balance of minerals in the body affects the metabolism, therefore a general mineral deficiency may predispose to laminitis.

3) High doses of steroids (cortisone) increase the response of

the digital blood vessels to circulating levels of adrenalin. This may result in 'shunting' and reduced blood flow to the foot.

The condition may be further complicated by secondary factors which include:

4) Sporadic intravascular coagulation — the pooling blood may clot in places, which further impedes the blood flow.

5) Changes in the levels of hormones produced by the endocrine glands. Marked changes in the levels of hormones including cortisol, testosterone, aldosterone, oestrogen, progesterone, renin and thyroxine could render the horse more susceptible to laminitis.

Treatment

Because of the serious nature of this ailment, the vet must be called for all but the mildest cases of laminitis. Mild may be interpreted as the signs being spotted and treated very quickly (same day) followed by rapid improvement (next day) and no reccurrence. Treatment may be divided into three categories:

1) Removal of the primary cause.
   (i) In the case of the grass-kept horse, he must be stabled on deep, non-edible bedding and fed only low feed value hay and water. Obese animals should have their food intake reduced gradually to avoid liver damage. A mineral supplement may be given. The vet may provide a specially formulated supplement or advise as to the type of supplement one should purchase. Alternatively a mineral lick should be available at all times.

   (The school of thought at one time was to feed bran mashes. This is now known to interfere further with the calcium:phosphorous ratio. Bran contains a high level of phosphorous and bran fibre inhibits the horse's ability to utilize calcium. Whenever bran, or indeed any grain, is fed, limestone flour should be added to boost calcium levels.)

   (ii) In the event of any infection, the vet will prescribe and administer the necessary antibiotics. If an infection is suspected, particularly in connection with a brood mare, the vet must be called immediately. (If the afterbirth has not come away within six hours, call the vet, who will administer oxytocin.)

(iii) If the horse has eaten a large quantity of feed, perhaps as a result of escaping and gorging in the feed room, the vet may administer a solution of liquid paraffin and electrolytes via a stomach tube as a bulk laxative, in order to clear out the system.

(iv) A supplement high in methionine should be given to re-establish the depleted keratin sulphate of the laminae.

2) Correction of circulation.
(i) The high blood pressure is partially a result of the great pain so, for the comfort of the horse, relief from pain must be a priority. The vet will prescribe an analgesic such as phenylbutazone; although research carried out has shown that this can affect the metabolism of sodium and potassium it is still the number one choice. (Bute must only be administered to ponies under veterinary prescription. It is known to cause liver damage and other side-effects in certain breeds of pony.) In endotoxaemic cases, a non-steroid anti-inflammatory drug such as flunixin may be given intravenously, followed by oral administration. Corticosteroid anti-inflammatories are contra-indicated as, for reasons unknown, they can actually *cause* laminitis and may make the situation worse. However, a single dose of cortisone may be administered intravenously on one day only. It is obviously important to be guided by the vet on current treatments for laminitis.
(i) Another form of treatment which may be used is a drug to reduce blood pressure, thus easing the congestion within the foot. Such a drug will need regular administration. Vasodilators (drugs which widen the blood vessels) are now being used and in some cases proving beneficial. Anticoagulant therapy has also been used. Careful monitoring of clotting ability is essential.

Hosing or tubbing with *warm* water will help to relax and dilate the capillaries within the foot, so easing congestion. However, another traditional treatment, now known to generally aggravate the condition, is cold hosing. The application of cold water causes further vasconstriction, impeding circulation. Nonetheless, in the very acute stage, cold hosing may assist insofar as it reduces the metabolic rate of the cells and thus reduces the tissues' demand for oxygen.

(ii) If there are no signs of pedal bone rotation, that is, if the laminitis is of the mildest form, gentle walking in hand can be practiced. The walking will improve circulation, but must be carried out on a soft surface. Exercise in the acute stage is recommended by most vets if there are no signs of pedal bone rotation, and if it does not exacerbate the pain. However, if there are any indications that the pedal bone has started to rotate (the horse shows signs of pain upon pressure on the sole or the laminitis is beyond the very mild stage), the walking exercise would cause further tearing of the laminae, and pain. This pain would aggravate the high blood pressure and the further damage to the laminae would cause greater rotation of the pedal bone. Therefore, in more severe cases box rest will encourage the damaged laminitic tissue to repair, so preventing further rotation.

3) Prevention of pedal bone rotation.
   If the laminitis is at all prolonged (signs persist for longer than a few days), it will be essential to have the feet x-rayed to determine whether the pedal bone has rotated and, if so, by how much. Only then can the vet and farrier plan a suitable programme of foot care. The most important factor to be considered when trying to prevent further rotation is that of resuming normal circulation. Having taken all of the necessary steps, the vet will advise as to the shoeing requirements of the laminitic horse.

   Once the stage of acute laminitis has passed, farriery can be carried out. The wall of the hoof will have to be cut back and the heel rasped down so as to realign the contours of the hoof to the new position of the pedal bone. Heart-bar shoes offer support to the pedal bone and take the pressure away from the toe, thus enabling the reattachment process to proceed unhindered. The heart-bar shoe must be accurately fitted. There must be a small gap between the ground surface of the frog and the 'V' section of the shoe to allow frog movement.

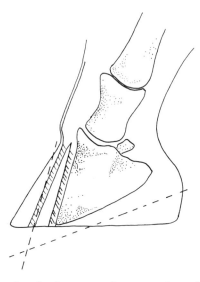

Figure 33 Corrective farriery to reduce rotation of the pedal bone

The broken lines show the desired contours of the wall — realigned with the new position of the pedal bone.

THE LYMPHATIC SYSTEM

The lymphatic system is closely integrated with the circulation of blood and consists of a network of blind-ended vessels running parallel to the blood vessels and permeating throughout the body tissues. The functions of the lymphatic system are:

To help return excess tissue fluid to blood.

To absorb and transport fats.

To filter out bacteria in lymph nodes.

To produce and store lymphocytes and antibodies.

The lymph vessels are tiny, blind-ending tubes which have very thin walls to allow the life-giving substances carried by lymph to diffuse through to the surrounding tissues and back again. Lymph is a transparent, yellow coloured fluid — it is basically plasma but with a lower proportion of proteins and glucose. Fat droplets are carried in this watery medium from chyle in the digestive tract to the liver. Waste products such as bacteria, debris and dead cells are also transported through the lymphatic system before being returned to the bloodstream prior to excretion.

The lymph vessels are similar to veins in that they have valves which ensure that the lymph is directed towards a vein. At intervals along these vessels are lymph nodes, bean-shaped tissue masses which act as filters against bacteria. They do this by containing stationary macrophages which engulf passing bacteria. Lymph nodes also produce lymphocytes and antibodies to fight infection. These nodes are grouped together to form lymph glands which may become swollen if the horse has an infection. These glands may be particularly noticeable under the jaw and in the throat area.

The lymphatic system has no motivating source of its own — it relies upon muscular activity to ensure the free flow of lymph. This explains why, in periods of enforced inactivity, the horse may be prone to puffy, fluid-filled legs. In extreme cases, when a dietary imbalance is also involved, the hind legs may be very hot and swollen, as occurs with the condition lymphangitis.

Disorders of the lymphatic system

Lymphangitis

Sporadic lymphangitis is also known as 'big leg' and 'Monday morning disease'.

Signs
A very swollen, warm hind limb. The horse shows signs of pain, which may include sweating, blowing, increased temperature and pulse rate.

Causes

1) It is not a common ailment and is thought to be caused by a metabolic imbalance, very similar to the factors which predispose azoturia. This imbalance may be brought about by enforced confinement on the normal corn diet.

2) Infection may cause inflammation and engorgement of the lymphatic vessels. A small cut may be found upon examination of the limb.

Treatment

Clean and treat any wound found.

Call the vet, who may administer anti-inflammatory, painkilling and antibiotic drugs.

Provide a low energy diet, such as bran mash and meadow hay. Add limestone flour to the bran mash to boost calcium levels.

Give vitamin and mineral supplements as advised by the vet.

Apply warm fomentations to the affected limb. Upward massage and bandaging (using ample gamgee as padding) will minimize swelling.

Gentle walking in hand will promote circulation. Often, walking is the only way to reduce swelling — it may have to be enforced.

Epizootic and ulcerative lymphangitis

These ailments affect horses abroad and are infections of the lymphatic system leading to inflammation and the formation of nodules which ultimately develop into ulcers, visible on the skin. Ulcerative lymphangitis is treated with antibiotics whilst epizootic lymphangitis is not normally considered worth treating, so the animal is destroyed. These conditions do not occur in Great Britain.

6

THE RESPIRATORY
SYSTEM

The functions of the respiratory system are:

Upon inhalation, to draw into the lungs air, which supplies oxygen, a gas essential for life.

Within the lungs, to transfer the oxygen from the air into the bloodstream.

To transfer carbon dioxide, the waste product of energy production, from the bloodstream to the lungs.

To expel carbon dioxide upon exhalation.

There are two types of respiration:

External respiration (breathing) is the transfer of gases between the external environment and the blood, and takes place within the airways of the head and neck and the lungs.

Cell, tissue or internal respiration is the metabolic breakdown of organic compounds, mainly carbohydrates, which occurs throughout the cells of the body, resulting in the release of energy.

Oxygen is normally required for the chemical reactions necessary for maintaining life. These reactions are controlled by enzymes. Once the energy has been released, the end products are carbon dioxide and water. Oxygen is transferred from the blood to all cells and carbon dioxide is transferred from these cells to the blood.

THE ANATOMY OF THE RESPIRATORY SYSTEM

The respiratory system consists of the airways (upper respiratory tract) and the bronchi and lungs (lower respiratory tract).

THE AIRWAYS

The nostrils. Air is drawn in through the nostrils; the horse is unable to breath in through his mouth.

The nasal cavities. These contain the turbinate bones which are covered with mucous membranes which warm and clean the incoming air. Tiny hairlike cilia project from these membranes and trap dust particles. The warmed air passes on to the pharynx.

The pharynx. This chamber at the back of the throat is used by both the respiratory and digestive systems. A musculo-membranous partition, the soft palate, separates the two systems' entrances into this chamber. The epiglottis overlaps the soft palate. During the process of breathing, it allows air to pass through to the larynx. When the horse swallows food, the epiglottis covers the larynx and the soft palate moves up to allow the food to pass into the oesophagus without interfering with the breathing process.

The larynx. This complex mechanism is situated at the top of the trachea and consists of interconnected cartilages, muscles and fibrous tissues covered by mucous membrane. Among these fibrous tissues are the vocal cords which, when vibrated by the forced passage of air, create sounds. The function of the larynx, apart from that of producing the voice, is to ensure that only gases pass into the deeper regions of the respiratory system; the larynx closes as soon as food particles touch the pharynx.

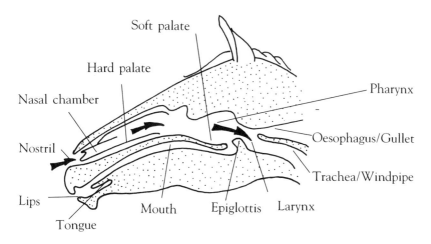

Figure 34 The anatomy of the upper respiratory tract

The trachea or windpipe, extends from the larynx down to the lungs and is held permanently open by rings of cartilage. Close to the lungs, the trachea branches into the two bronchi. The trachea is lined by millions of tiny hairs, cilia, which assist in removing mucus by their wavelike motion.

THE LOWER RESPIRATORY TRACT

The bronchi. These tubes are held open by thin rings of cartilage and each enter one lung, where they then continue to divide, forming a bronchial 'tree'. The branches get progressively smaller, the narrowest being known as bronchioles (see Figure 35).

The bronchioles. These very narrow tubes are lined with a continuation of the ciliated mucous membrane and are not supported by cartilaginous rings. The smallest of the bronchioles are known as respiratory bronchioles, each of which then further divide into alveolar ducts.

The alveoli at the end of each duct are the air sacs which make up the lung tissue. There are millions of thin-walled alveoli, giving a huge surface area — estimated at several hundred square metres. In order to keep the airways moist, a thin film of mucus is secreted by cells lining the alveoli. In a healthy horse the mucus never accumulates to a serious degree.

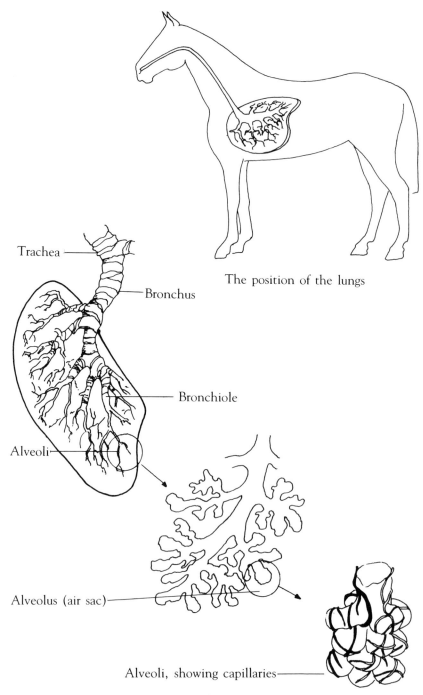

The position of the lungs

Trachea

Bronchus

Bronchiole

Alveoli

Alveolus (air sac)

Alveoli, showing capillaries

Figure 35 The anatomy of the lower respiratory tract

Permeating through the alveoli are the capillaries of the pulmonary artery. It is here that the gaseous exchange occurs.

The outer surface of the lung tissue is covered by the pleura — a serous (smooth, moist) membrane that also lines the thoracic cavity and allows the lungs to slide freely within this cavity.

Gaseous exchange

The thin film of liquid secreted by the alveoli also acts as a medium for diffusion. The deoxygenated blood in the capillaries is very close to the surface of the alveoli. The carbon dioxide within this blood diffuses into the air in the alveoli and is expelled when the horse breathes out.

Oxygen diffuses from the air into the alveoli, through the thin capillary walls, and combines with the haemoglobin in the blood.

EXTERNAL RESPIRATION

External respiration consists of breathing in (inhalation or inspiration) and breathing out (exhalation or expiration).

Inhalation occurs as a result of expansion of the rib cage, which causes the dome-shaped diaphragm (the muscular sheet dividing the chest from the belly) to contract and flatten, so enlarging the thorax and reducing the air pressure within the lungs to below that of the external environment. This difference in pressure causes air to be pulled into the respiratory system through the nostrils, thus increasing the pressure in the lungs. As the ribs recoil to their original position, so the diaphragm relaxes and returns to its dome-shaped position.

Exhalation occurs as the chest volume decreases and the pressure within the thoracic cavity increases, forcing air out of the lungs. Exhalation is mainly a passive process but the trunk muscles can assist by pushing the gut contents against the diaphragm. The diaphragm begins just in front of the loins and slopes downwards and forwards to the breastbone. The oesophagus and major blood vessels pass through the diaphragm into the abdominal cavity.

INTERNAL (TISSUE) RESPIRATION

Internal respiration occurs when the oxygen in the blood (oxyhaemoglobin) reaches the body tissue. Every vital activity of the cells requires energy. A series of chemical reactions causes energy to be produced from glucose in the blood or glycogen in muscle cells.

Within every cell are high-energy compounds called adenosine triphosphate (ATP). Each compound consists of a complex organic molecule of adenosine to which is attached a chain of three phosphate groups. In the presence of the correct enzyme, one of the phosphate groups is broken off, an action which releases a large amount of free energy. Some of this energy is lost as heat but the remainder (mechanical energy) can be used directly for biological activities.

Once the energy has been released the ATP compound becomes ADP — adenosine diphosphate (adenosine to which are attached two phosphate groups). ADP has then to be regenerated back to ATP; this occurs quickly. The rate at which ATP is re-formed must correspond with the rate at which the original ATP is broken down to provide energy. Therefore the harder the horse is working, the faster this regeneration must occur.

During tissue respiration, sugars are broken down to provide the energy for the regeneration of ATP. Simplified, this occurs when a phosphate group is attached to the ADP. This regeneration of ATP and the release of energy when ATP is converted to ADP take place within the mitochondria, sausage-shaped structures referred to as the powerhouses of a cell. On average each cell contains about 1,000 mitochondria.

The rate at which sugar is broken down depends upon the amount of ATP being used up. Very little ATP is stored within the cell — the horse's metabolism ensures that it is regenerated at the same rate as it is needed. When this metabolism occurs in the presence of oxygen it is referred to as aerobic metabolism or respiration, the end products of which are carbon dioxide and water. The carbon dioxide attaches to the haemoglobin in the blood and is carried to the lungs, from where it is expelled.

During prolonged, strenuous exercise the demands of the body may not be met fully by the oxygen arriving in the blood. In this instance, the respiration takes place without oxygen, that is, by anaerobic respiration. However, this process is less efficient; the sugars are only partially broken down, resulting in the production of less energy and a potentially harmful end product, lactic acid, which is removed in the bloodstream and transported to the liver for detoxification.

When lactic acid is oxygenated it is reconverted to sugars, any acid not reconverted being broken down and excreted. Anaerobic respiration is therefore, a useful — sometimes essential — short-term means of energy production.

A problem can arise, however, if a build-up of lactic acid reduces the pH of the cell to an extent at which the cell becomes too acid: ATP cannot be produced efficiently, which results in fatigue. The muscle fibres cannot contract properly and normal functioning is impaired, giving rise to cramp-like symptoms (tying-up syndrome) and/or muscle fatigue. It is, therefore, undesirable to work a horse strenuously beyond his level of fitness for any length of time.

Oxygen is essential for the removal of lactic acid so, after strenuous work, the horse will 'blow' for much longer as his lungs strive to draw in air and so pay off the 'oxygen debt' which has arisen as a result of prolonged anaerobic respiration.

THE EFFECT OF WORK UPON THE RESPIRATORY SYSTEM

The normal rate of breaths per minute in the adult horse at rest is between eight and sixteen. Youngstock have a slightly higher rate. During strenuous exercise the rate may increase to 120 breaths per minute in order to cope with the body's extra oxygen requirements. At canter and gallop, the respiratory rate is locked to the stride rate.

One aim of fitness work with any horse is, among other things, to increase his ability to supply and utilize oxygen. The unfit horse does not have so great a functional lung capacity as a fit one because not all of the alveoli are recruited. Upon exercise of an unfit horse there may be a slight nasal discharge. This may result from a sub-clinical infection causing an enlargement of the lymph follicles in the lining of the throat.

As fitness progresses so more alveoli become clear, thus increasing the amount of functional area available for gaseous exchange. This is known as alveolar recruitment. As the surface area of useful lung tissue increases, so the capillaries surrounding the alveoli proliferate. This pulmonary capillarization provides a greater surface area for the increased gaseous exchange necessary in the working horse.

As the horse's general fitness improves, so his muscles will develop. This will include the muscles of the diaphragm and chest, further aiding efficient breathing.

DISORDERS OF THE RESPIRATORY SYSTEM

Respiratory disorders can vary from a mild nasal discharge which has no other adverse effects on the horse's health if dealt with promptly, to a severely debilitating viral infection.

Signs which suggest that all is not right may include any combination of the following:

Nasal discharge — colour and viscosity will vary according to the condition.

Coughing — may vary from a soft, wet cough to a harsh, dry one which may be persistent or occur only when the horse is working.

Generally dull attitude, loss of performance and weight loss.

Respiratory distress after exercise.

Swollen glands around the throat.

Rise in temperature — may be slight or as high as 106 °F (41 °C.)

Causes of respiratory disease

Viruses. The most common cause of respiratory disease is one of the many types of virus. Viruses are micro-organisms so small they cannot be seen using a normal microscope. They exist throughout the environment but being parasitic cannot multiply unless living within a host cell. Viruses may attack the mucosa of the nasal passages and airways, and use the energy and materials of these cells to multiply by replication. As the virus multiplies so the host cells are killed.

Bacteria. Bacteria are minute, single-celled living organisms which are large enough to be seen under a normal light microscope. An example of a respiratory tract disorder caused by bacteria would be strangles, which is caused by Streptococcus equi.

The subject of viruses and bacteria will be discussed more fully further on (Chapter 8).

Internal parasites. Lungworms (Dictyocaulus arnfieldi) cause considerable damage to the lungs throughout their life cycle. External signs are coughing and nasal discharge.

Dust. Inhaled dust particles will irritate the sensitive mucous membranes of the airways. Dust from bedding, hay and working surfaces are great contributors to repiratory problems.

Fungal spores. Hay and straw often harbour fungal spores which, once inhaled, irritate the respiratory system and may trigger an allergic response.

Mites and mite faeces. Mites are pests harboured in some stored feed. Old, stale feed provides the ideal breeding ground for mites.

The effects of disease upon the respiratory tract

Excess mucus production. The airways are lined with mucous membranes, the secretions of which help to trap dust particles or bacteria which may then be transported to the throat from where they are swallowed. They are later excreted via the digestive tract.

As a result of excessive debris and/or the invasion of bacteria, the mucus becomes thicker and stickier. It is then far more difficult for the horse to shift, with the result that the bronchioles become blocked. This reduces the capacity for gaseous exchange, so the horse is unable to breath and work efficiently.

Coughing. The cough is triggered by irritation of the airways and helps to shift the sticky mucus. If the ailment is infectious, the coughing process leads to widespread dispersal of infectious bacteria or viruses.

Restriction of airways. The muscular walls of the airways contract in response to irritation from dust particles, bacteria etc. When disease is present, the muscle becomes very sensitive and over-constricted. This condition, which restricts the free passage of air, is known as bronchospasm. Any air which passes through the much-restricted airways may rush through more quickly, possibly causing a wheezing noise as it does so.

Inflammation. The excessive irritation leads to a sensitive, inflamed state of the lining of the airways. This inflammation causes narrowing of the airways, which again restricts airflow.

INFECTIONS OF THE UPPER RESPIRATORY TRACT

Cold or chill

Signs
Clear nasal discharge which later thickens, becoming whitish in colour.

Cough.

Swollen glands around the throat and difficulty in swallowing.

Slight rise in temperature.

Causes

Viral infection which may take hold whilst horse is vulnerable, for example in a badly ventilated, draughty stable or lorry; stabled initially after living out at grass; run-down horse in a generally poor condition.

Treatment

Call the vet, who may take nasal swabs for a more positive diagnosis. He may also listen to the lungs with the stethoscope to help verify that the infection is mainly affecting the upper respiratory tract.

Isolate and rest horse and adhere to relevant rules of sick nursing: warmth, fresh air, (but no draughts), damp, soft food and complete rest.

Inhalations of Friar's Balsam may help to clear the airways.

Strangles

This highly contagious condition affects the upper respiratory tract and is caused by the bacteria Streptococcus equi. The source of infection is either a diseased animal, inhalation of infective air or contact with infected woodwork (the bacteria found in pus from a strangles abscess may remain infective within a structure for many months).

Signs

The incubation period (period between becoming infected and showing the first signs) is generally between three and six days. The first sign is disinterest in taking food or water. This is followed by:

A thick nasal discharge of pus-like appearance.

Coughing.

A rise in temperature, which may go as high as 106 °F (41 °C).

The lymph glands in the throat region become swollen and the horse may experience difficulty in swallowing.

The horse may stand with his neck distended.

Abscesses may form at the site of the lymph glands. These will eventually mature, burst and drain.

Treatment

Adhere to strict isolation rules and call the vet, who may take swabs from nasal discharge or pus from abscesses to test for Streptococci equi.

Antibiotics, in particular penicillin, are effective against these bacteria. Early, prompt and continued treatment may prevent abscess formation. However, in the later stages of this condition, antibiotic therapy may delay the maturing and bursting of the abscesses. In such instances, antibiotics may be withheld until the abscesses have ruptured.

Hot fomentation of abscesses will help them to mature — once mature they may be surgically drained. At this point the healing process is more noticeable as the horse starts to show signs of recovery. Remove purulent discharges with non-irritating antiseptic solution.

The vet may administer non-steroid anti-inflammatory drugs to reduce the pain and improve the appetite. However, while the horse is unwell, feed only soft mashes.

As this condition is often severely debilitating, the horse will need a very long period of rest.

In a more chronic form, the condition is known as bastard strangles — it is not epidemic, affecting only individual horses. The signs include fever, and abscesses which may appear in different areas of the body.

Laryngitis and tracheitis

These are infections of the upper respiratory tract which cause inflammation of the larynx or trachea. They may occur singly or together.

Signs

Difficulty in swallowing.

Laboured breathing.

Coughing.

Rise in temperature.

Nasal discharge.

Cause
Bacterial infection.

Treatment
Call the vet, who may administer antibiotics.

Damp all feed well — give mashes and gruels.

Keep the horse warm, but ensure plenty of fresh air and follow general rules of sick nursing.

Laryngeal paralysis (whistling and roaring)

Signs
Whistling and roaring are abnormal inspiratory sounds heard when the horse canters and gallops. They result from air rushing past a paralysed cartilage and vocal cord in the larynx. Whistling is a high pitched sound whilst roaring is much lower pitched. Both are heard during inspiration.

Whistling and roaring must not be confused with 'high blowing', which is simply a vibration of the false nostril while the horse works, not an ailment or unsoundness. No inspiratory noise is heard in a normal horse.

Causes
The larynx consists of a cartilagenous tube. On either side of its roof are the arytenoid cartilages. Extending downwards to the floor of the larynx are the vocal cords, made up of fibrous cords and ventricles (membranous folds).

When the horse is at rest the vocal cords hang inwards, but during exercise, muscular contractions cause the arytenoid cartilages to be pulled outwards which, in turn, pulls the vocal cords to the side thus opening the airway and allowing a free flow of inspired air.

Whistling and roaring are signs of laryngeal paralysis; as a result of degeneration of the nerve supplying the abductor muscle on the left side of the larynx, the left vocal cord is not pulled out of the way. The sounds are caused by the turbulent air trying to flow past the obstruction. The degeneration of the nerve supply may occur following respiratory tract diseases such as strangles, bronchitis, influenza and pharyngitis. However, it is particularly common in large and well grown horses and it is thought that hereditary tendencies may also be involved.

Treatment

If the horse is able to perform his required level of work without respiratory distress, no action will be needed. However, if the obstruction is severe, the horse's capacity for fast work will be impaired. Examination by endoscope (a fibre-optic device which is inserted into the respiratory tract) will enable the vet to assess the degree of paralysis. Muscle wastage is assessed by palpation of the throat from the outside. The vet can then take one of the following courses of action:

Hobdaying is a simple operation whereby the laryngeal ventricle is removed under general anaesthetic. A horse who has been hobdayed is not allowed to compete in show hunter classes.

'Tie back'. An alternative or addition to hobdaying is the laryngeal prothesis operation, sometimes referred to as 'tie back'. The left arytenoid cartilage is stitched back so that the vocal cord is permanently open, allowing free flow of air through the larynx.

Tubing (tracheotomy) is the insertion of a tube into the trachea just below the larynx, allowing air to be inhaled in a way that bypasses the obstruction.

Provided that there are no secondary complications, horses who have undergone these processes may lead completely normal lives. The one exception is that any form of hydrotherapy would be impractical in the case of a tubed horse because of the possibility of him inhaling large quantities of water — even drowning. The stable environment for such horses must be kept as free from dust as possible; bedding or hay should not be shaken up near a tubed horse.

Sinusitis

This is an infection within one of the sinuses, causing inflammation of the membranous lining and the accumulation of pus.

Although the sinuses are not directly involved in the process of respiration, their infection may be secondary to respiratory disorder and signs are closely associated to those of the upper respiratory tract.

Signs
Greyish nasal discharge, normally from one nostril.

Swollen, tender area around sinus – normally just beneath the eye.

Causes
1) Bacterial infection secondary to a cold, strangles, or similar.

2) Infection arising from a damaged tooth root.

Treatment
The vet may drain the sinus and administer antibiotics.

INFECTIONS OF THE LOWER RESPIRATORY TRACT

Equine influenza

Over the years the transportation of horses around the world has become more practical and affordable, particularly for those involved in competition, racing and sales. With the horse population travelling greater distances both at home and abroad, the risk of spreading infectious diseases increases.

Equine influenza is a highly contagious disease caused by various strains and sub-types of flu virus. Continuing research means that further sub-types of virus may be identified. The two main types of virus are Myxovirus A/Equi 1 (Prague 56) – a virus which has been around for decades, and Myxovirus A/Equi 2 (Miami 63). The latter was first recognized in 1963 and is particularly harmful, killing foals and yearlings and causing permanent lung damage in older horses. These two strains of virus produce different antigens so can be separately identified.

Signs
General lethargy, dullness and loss of appetite.

Sharp rise in temperature, up to 105−107°F (40.5−41.5°C).

Frequent, dry cough lasting two to three weeks or even longer.

Nasal discharge which is initially clear and watery, but becomes thicker and pus-like as the disease progresses.

Difficulty in breathing.

There may be difficulty in swallowing and swollen glands.

Equine influenza spreads rapidly through a yard as each cough expels large quantities of infective virus into the air, which is then inhaled by other horses. The incubation period is extremely short, ranging from one to five days − the horse may begin to show signs as early as twenty-four hours after initial infection. The horse remains infectious for between six and ten days after the onset of signs.

Treatment
Call the vet, who may administer antibiotics to prevent any secondary complications caused by bacteria. He may also send a swab of discharge and/or a blood sample to the laboratory for analysis to determine the exact strain of 'flu or to check whether the signs are a result of infection by the equine herpes virus − equine viral rhinopneumonitis (EHV-1).

Adhere to all rules of isolation and sick nursing. Stringent precautions must be taken to ensure good stable hygiene. There are now specially prepared stable and yard disinfectants on the market which are effective against bacteria and viruses.

Ensure a dust-free environment and very good ventilation.

After an attack, a long period of rest is essential; mildly affected animals may recover in two to three weeks, but those severely affected may need as long as six months to convalesce. It is extremely important that horses are not put back into work until completely recovered. As a general rule, for every day that the horse's temperature is raised above normal − 100.5°F (38°C) − he will need one week of complete rest.

There is always a risk of secondary conditions such as emphysema, chronic bronchitis and bacterial pneumonia occurring.

This risk will be greatly increased if the horse returns to work too soon because the influenza virus also damages heart muscle and liver tissue. This may lead to impaired circulation and jaundice.

Prevention
1) Keep all horses fully inoculated. This practice is required by all major showgrounds and racecourses, whilst registration of horses with many groups, for example the BHS Horse Trials Group, is subject to the horse having a fully completed, up-to-date vaccination certificate. Under Jockey Club rules, the primary vaccination course or booster injections must be given at least ten clear days prior to attending a racecourse.

2) Isolate all new horses as they enter the yard — particularly those from overseas or the sale ring. Bearing in mind that the incubation period is between one and five days, the horse should remain segregated for this length of time.

3) Similarly, minimize the risk of contact with strange horses; do not allow your animals to come into very close contact with others at shows, meets etc.

4) Foals born to fully vaccinated mares will receive antibodies via the mare's colostrum. This will protect the foal for the first three months of his life, after which he will require vaccination. Foals born to unvaccinated mares should be vaccinated earlier than three months of age, as should any foal who may be at risk of infection during an epidemic.

Vaccination
Primary Vaccination. Jockey Club rules state that the first two influenza injections should be given not less than twenty-one days and not more than ninety-two days apart. In order to comply with this, the first two injections are given four to six weeks apart. 150−215 days after the second injection, a third is given, completing the primary course of vaccination.

Following the primary vaccinations, the horse should not be subjected to severe exertion; exercise should be light for at least seven days. This is because the vaccine may give rise to a slight reaction which would be aggravated by strenuous exercise.

Boosters. The first booster is given six months after completion of the primary course and from then on normally every nine to twelve months. The higher the risk of infection, the more frequently the horse should receive a booster.

Following booster vaccinations, light work must be maintained for two to three days.

Equine viral rhinopneumonitis (EVR)

This condition, which is caused by the equine herpes virus 1 (EHV-1), of which there are two sub types, primarily produces respiratory catarrh. It is often seen in foals, particularly those in areas of dense equine population such as studs. The Horserace Betting Levy Board has prepared a Code of Practice for the United Kingdom and Ireland with regard to all aspects of EHV-1. If EHV-1 is confirmed, the appropriate breeders' association should be informed.

Signs
The incubation period is between two and ten days.

Temperature will rise to between 102 and 107 °F (39−41.5 °C), for a period of between one and seven days.

Leucopenia − a drop in white blood cell count.

Congestion and serous discharge from nasal mucosa and conjunctiva.

Disinterest in food, water and a generally dull appearance.

Cough.

In some cases the horse will suffer from pharyngitis and swollen glands in the throat region.

Sometimes constipation is followed by diarrhoea.

Certain outbreaks are seen to affect the central nervous system, causing a lack of co-ordination and possibly paralysis of the hindquarters.

When pregnant mares are affected, they may abort approximately three to four weeks after infection (usually in the last trimester). The abortion is sudden, followed by prompt expulsion of the placenta, or the foetus may be delivered in the membranes. The future breeding capacity of the mare is not normally impaired.

Causes
The virus may remain dormant within an infected horse, who appears to be completely normal. There is no test to detect latent carriers. The virus may be activated by stress. The disease is then transmitted through either direct or indirect contact with infective nasal discharge, aborted foetuses or placentas. Foals infected in the first manner will carry and spread the virus for up to nine days while appearing normal. Foals infected neonatally (within the uterus) invariably die.

Treatment
Call the vet as soon as initial signs are noticed. Nasal swabs may be taken to give positive identification of the virus. Any aborted foetus and placenta should be sent for post-mortem examination.

Adhere to strict rules of isolation. Steam clean and disinfect any affected stable and burn all bedding.

Prevent all movement of horses in and out of the yard. Keep all other stock away from pregnant mares.

A detailed description of this disease and its control in breeding stock is given in another book in this series — *The Horse: Breeding and Youngstock*.

Immunity
The horse will acquire a certain degree of immunity following infection. A live vaccine may be administered although, where breeding stock is concerned, it is usual to use a killed vaccine for fear of reversion to virulence. Pregnant mares may be administered killed viral vaccine in the fifth, seventh and ninth months of pregnancy to help prevent abortions. The subject of live and dead vaccines is dealt with later (The Sick Horse). All horses on the premises should be vaccinated as a preventative measure.

Bronchitis

This is an inflammatory condition which normally affects the bronchi but can affect the bronchioles — in which case it is known as bronchiolitis. Very often these conditions are secondary to another infection. If they result from bacterial or viral infection, the disease may be transmitted. Any infection and/or dust etc. can cause bronchitis as part of the disease process; it is part of many disease conditions affecting the respiratory tract.

Signs
Coughing spasms — the cough may persist for two to three weeks.

Bilateral nasal discharge.

A slight rise in temperature.

A generally dull, depressed state.

When the bronchitis is caused through bacterial infection, examination by endoscope may show mucopurulent exudate in the trachea.

Causes
As mentioned above, these may include: bacterial or viral infection; allergens; the inhalation of smoke or irritant gases; the presence of foreign bodies in the airways.

Treatment
The vet may administer antibiotics to treat bacterial infection, and also mucolytic drugs (which aid the breakdown and clearance of mucus).

Adhere to the general rules of sick nursing; complete rest, plenty of fresh air, a dust-free environment. Keep the horse warm and feed soft, easily swallowed and digestible food.

Pneumonia

This serious condition causes inflammation of the lungs and bronchi. Foals, especially those under six months old are particularly susceptible to bacterial pneumonia and may become very ill.

Signs
Coughing.

An increase in temperature − possibly to 107 °F (41.5 °C).

Increased rate of pulse and respiration.

Mucopurulent discharge in trachea and at nostrils.

The horse will appear very cold and tucked up, with poor appetite.

Causes
Bacterial, viral or fungal infection.

Parasitic damage.

Pneumonia may also occur as a secondary infection to equine influenza or, particularly in foals, inherited immuno-deficiency.

Treatment
Immediately seek and follow veterinary advice. The vet may administer a combination of antibiotics, bronchodilators and mucolytics.

Keep the horse warm − with rugs and possibly heat lamps and provide plenty of draught-free fresh air.

Epistaxis (nosebleed)

Epistaxis is not an actual disease, but a clinical sign that underlying problems exist.

Signs
Blood may pour down either one or both nostrils. Bleeding from both nostrils indicates haemorrhage of the lungs, whilst bleeding from one nostril may be an indication of problems in the pharynx or guttural pouch.

Causes
1) The stress of racing causes bleeding from the smallest vessels in the lungs (exercise-induced pulmonary haemorrhage).

The horse is often described as having 'broken blood vessels'. The bleeding, originating from the lungs, may occur from both nostrils. (It is thought that *some* bleeding occurs in all racehorses — only if it is severe will it be seen from the nostrils.)

2) Guttural pouch mycosis — a serious fungal condition affecting the pouch, possibly leading to an aneurism of the carotid artery in the roof of the guttural pouch. Haemorrhage from the guttural pouch can be so profuse that death may result.

3) Pharyngeal abscess. This produces a bloody nasal discharge which may also contain food and pus. Other symptoms of this condition include difficulty in breathing and swallowing.

4) A fracture of the skull and/or bruising of the nasal cavity.

5) Small growths in the mucous membrane of the nasal cavity.

Treatment

If the bleeding is severe or the cause unknown, consult the vet.

Exercise-induced pulmonary haemorrhage (EIPH), occurs in racehorses as a result of high blood pressure in the small thin-walled capillary networks in the lungs. Diuretics such as frusemide have been administered in an attempt to eliminate excess fluid from the body and therefore reduce blood pressure. Also, Vitamins C and K may be added to the diet to aid the clotting of blood.

It should be noted, however, that Jockey Club and FEI rules do not permit actual competition whilst under medication.

Obstructive pulmonary disease (OPD)

This is a physiological description of a condition affecting the respiratory tract which, if not treated, may become chronic (COPD).

Signs

The initial changes which occur within the lower respiratory tract may not be noticed at first. These changes include:

Excessive mucus production.

Inflammation of the epithelia lining the airways.

Bronchospasm (spasm of the muscles lining the walls of the bronchi and the bronchioles).

The external symptoms include:

Coughing — both at rest and during work, which may be aggravated by exercise.

Mucopus, discharged from the nostrils, found on the stable door or yard each morning.

Increased resting respiratory rate.

Reduced performance.

Causes
The condition is often, but not always, allergic in origin; inhalation of dust particles and fungal spores causes an allergic reaction. Other possible contributory factors are:

Foreign bodies causing lesions of the upper airways.

Parasitic damage (for example lungworm, especially if there is contact with donkeys).

Bronchitis/bronchiolitis.

The condition may also occur secondary to a viral infection.

Treatment
Ensure a dust-free environment (see later). If all else appears normal:

Worm, using ivermectin, an anthelmintic which is effective against lungworm.

If other clinical signs (rise in temperature, loss of appetite etc.) are evident, or those present persist, call the vet who may administer one or a combination of the following drugs:

Bronchodilators. These are drugs which cause the restricted muscles of the airways to relax, so reducing the bronchospasm and allowing a freer flow of air. The bronchodilator commonly in use is clenbuterol, marketed as Ventipulmin, which may be administered in feed or by injection.

Anti-inflammatories. These are administered either orally or intravenously, and may include drugs such as steroids and non-steroidal anti-inflammatories such as flunixin meglumine (marketed as Finadyne) or phenylbutazone.

Mucolytics. These drugs help to reduce the viscosity of the mucus by decreasing the protein content. They are usually administered orally in the form of powders taken in the feed.

Another treatment is nebulization. Drugs can be inhaled by the horse with the use of a special inhalation kit called a nebulizer. An example is the anti-allergy drug sodium cromo-glycate (marketed as Cromovet), which is converted into a fine mist by the nebulizer, then enters the mask and is inhaled to desensitize the allergic cells for a period of up to twenty days.

Chronic alveolar emphysema

Also known as 'broken winded' and 'heaves', this is a progressive condition for which there is no actual cure; good stable management may keep the horse's discomfort to a minimum.

Signs
Persistent, harsh cough.

Possible loss of condition and/or stamina.

Laboured exhalation.

There may be a nasal discharge.

Causes
The physiological damage is caused through interference in the free flow of air by obstructions in the airways. An obstruction such as bronchospasm (the muscles lining the bronchi walls go into spasm, thereby restricting the airway) will restrict the flow of used air being exhaled — this means that a new inhalation

may have started before all the air from the previous breath has been expelled. This leads to over-inflation of the alveoli, possibly resulting in damage to the thin alveolar walls. A double exhalatory effort is required to expel the used air, causing the muscles involved in this effort to become overdeveloped. The abdominal muscles become ridged, forming what is known as a 'heaves' or pleuritic line. Underlying causes are:

Obstructive pulmonary disease.

Allergic reaction to dust, moulds etc.

Extreme exertion when unfit.

The condition may be secondary to a bacterial or viral infection of the respiratory tract.

Treatment
Follow the advice of the vet; treat as for COPD to alleviate obstructed airways and keep the environment as dust-free as possible.

Take great care when working — keep well within the horse's capabilities. If the condition is very bad, he may only be capable of light work.

Provision of a dust-free environment

This is an important aspect of stable management for both allergic and non-allergic horses. Horses living out are much less prone to respiratory disorders because their environment is relatively free of dust and they are constantly breathing fresh air. It would, however, be impractical in most cases to expect a fit competition horse to live out permanently because of the difficulties in monitoring feed intake and maintenance of condition. Nonetheless, all horses benefit from a daily period spent out at grass, not only for the well-being of their respiratory systems, but also for their mental state.

While a horse is stabled, dust can be minimized by attention to the following:

Ventilation must be draught-free but substantial, ensuring at least six changes of air every hour.

Bedding. Always use shavings or shredded paper as bedding for an allergic horse and do not muck out while he is in the box. In adjoining stables which may share the same air space, be careful not to shake up a straw bed while the allergic horse is in residence next door. If possible, bed *all* horses on dust-free material.

Thorough mucking out is essential − the use of stable disinfectants will help prevent the build up of ammonia, the fumes of which are very irritating to the sensitive mucous membranes of the respiratory tract, and paralyse the cilia, so that mucus is not brought up the airway efficiently. Damp bedding is the ideal medium for fungal spores, so ensure bedding is always as dry as possible. Deep litter bedding would not be suitable for an allergic horse.

Stables need to be kept as free from cobwebs and dust as is possible.

Feeding. Use a machine such as the DustCure machine to remove excessive dust and debris from hay and straw. Feed soaked and/or steamed, good quality hay. Hosing under high pressure, or immersing for several minutes then draining has been proven to remove an optimum amount of dust and spores without reducing the nutrient value in the way that overnight soaking does. Horsehage or complete cubes are free from dust and spores.

Give all feeds well dampened. Molasses in the feed helps spores stick to the feedstuffs and ingestion is not harmful.

7

THE URINARY SYSTEM

The function of the urinary system is to remove excess water and unwanted substances from the body as urine. The main functional organs of the system are the kidneys; these produce the urine which is transported out of the body via the ureters, bladder and urethra.

ANATOMY OF THE URINARY SYSTEM

The kidneys

These are a pair of organs situated high up against the roof of the abdomen. Each kidney weighs approximately 700 grams (23 oz). The right kidney lies beneath the last two or three ribs and the first lumbar vertebra. The left kidney lies beneath the last rib and the first two or three lumbar vertebrae. The kidneys are held in place by the surrounding organs and dense fibrous connective tissue — renal fascia. Each kidney is enveloped in a fibrous coat of dense connective tissue known as the kidney capsule.

The renal nerves and artery enter the kidney at an indentation known as the hilus; the renal veins, lymphatic vessels and ureter leave the kidney at this point. The body of the kidney is composed of three main parts; the cortex, the medulla and the renal pelvis.

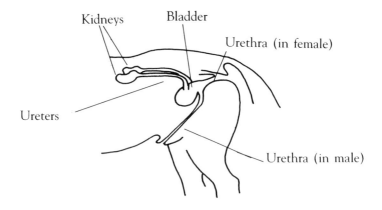

Figure 36 The organs of the urinary system

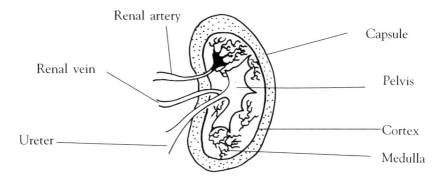

Figure 37 The structure of a kidney

The cortex

The outermost part of the kidney, the cortex, has a granular appearance and is coloured reddish-brown by many small dark spots known as malpighian corpuscles.

Most of the filtration of fluids occurs in the cortex. Within the cortex there are many thousands of minute filtration units known as kidney tubules (also referred to as renal tubules or nephrons). These are composed of:

The glomerulus — A small knot of blood vessels.

Bowman's capsule — A blind-ended tube which expands to sorround the glomerulus. The first stage of filtration occurs here.

Tubules — The point at which the tubule is nearest the Bowman's capsule is called the proximal tubule. This extends downwards to form the loop of Henle, beyond which is the distal tubule.

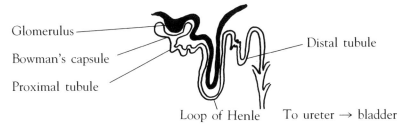

Glomerulus

Bowman's capsule

Proximal tubule

Distal tubule

Loop of Henle   To ureter → bladder

Figure 38 A kidney tubule

The medulla

This structure of deep red tissue lies within the outer cortex. After filtration, fluids from the tubules finally empty into collection ducts which converge to form papillary ducts within the medulla.

The renal pelvis

This is the collecting area for the urine arriving from the papillary ducts. The pelvis narrows dramatically and forms the ureter.

Other organs of the urinary system

The urinary functions started in the kidneys are completed by a complementary system consisting of:

The ureter

This tube extends backwards and downwards from the renal pelvis of the kidney to the neck of the bladder. Urine is passed through the ureter, which has a fibrous outer layer, muscular middle layer and is lined by a mucous membrane. Each kidney has its own ureter leading into the bladder. The urine is passed along the ureters through muscular contractions known as peristalsis.

The bladder

The outer layer of the bladder is covered by an incomplete peritoneal membrane which folds to form many attachments within the abdomen, holding the bladder in position.

The bladder is lined with a mucous membrane. The bladder wall is composed of fibrous tissue, rich in blood vessels. The fibres of the strong, muscular outer layer run in all directions except at the neck, where the fibres take a circular form to create a sphincter muscle.

When the bladder is full, sensory nerve impulses are transmitted to the central nervous system. In response, motor nerve impulses cause the bladder to contract and the sphincter muscle to relax, thus allowing the horse to urinate.

The urethra

This tube leads from the neck of the bladder to the outside. In the female the urethra is fairly short, opening into the floor of the vestibule within the vagina. In the male the urethra is much longer, extending downwards to the tip of the penis. It transports both urine and semen; the contractions of the muscular layers covering the urethra force these fluids along the tube.

FUNCTIONS OF THE KIDNEYS

The functions of the kidneys are:

1) To filter the water and unwanted substances including toxins from the blood.

The pressure within the blood vessels of the glomerulus is greater than that within the Bowman's capsule. The difference between the two pressures is called the filtration pressure and it is this which causes the constant passage of filtrate (renal filtration) between the glomerulus and renal tubules. Should infection be present in the body, the circulating toxins are filtered out in the normal way.

2) To reabsorb the correct balance of salts and fluid.

Once the filtering process is complete, regulated quantities of certain substances are reabsorbed according to the needs of the body. Some substances are totally readmitted into the bloodstream while others, such as urea and toxins, are only reabsorbed in minute quantities. This 'selective reabsorption helps:

3) To maintain a constant level of fluid within the body.

The amount of filtrate passed is dependent on the filtration pressure. This pressure is affected by the arterial pressure, that is, by anything causing a reduction in blood pressure. Haemorrhage, for example, will reduce the pressure within the glomerulus, thereby lowering the filtration pressure; the amount of filtrate passed is then also lowered. The consequence of this interaction is that, in the event of abnormal fluid loss or shock, the kidneys reduce the amount of fluid excreted as urine.

When arterial pressure is low the kidneys produce the enzyme renin which, in turn, converts one of the plasma proteins into angiotensin, a substance which causes the constriction of blood vessels, thus increasing blood pressure. Angiotensin also stimulates the cortex of the adrenal gland to produce the hormone aldosterone. Aldosterone favours the retention of sodium, and thus water, thereby playing a vital role in the maintenance of the volume of body fluids.

A high percentage of water is reabsorbed in the proximal tubules. In the distal tubules, sodium ions are reabsorbed or exchanged for hydrogen, potassium or ammonium ions. As the filtrate passes along the remainder of the renal tubule most of it is reabsorbed through the tubule wall into the surrounding tissue fluid, then into a network of adjacent capillaries. It is possible to increase the filtration rate, causing the production of more urine, through the dilation of the capillaries of the glomerulus. Substances used to achieve this effect are known as diuretics.

Located in the hypothalamus at the base of the pituitary gland is a group of osmoreceptor cells, sensitive to the osmotic pressure of the blood. These cells are stimulated by a rise in osmotic pressure, for example when the body becomes dehydrated or a large amount of salt is consumed. This triggers the release of the hormone vasopressin (ADH) which directs the kidneys to produce a more concentrated urine, therefore lowering the osmotic pressure. When the reverse occurs, for example after the horse has drunk large quantities of water, less hormone is produced, resulting in a more dilute urine being produced. This results in a rise in the osmotic pressure of the blood and tissue fluids.

4) To maintain the correct mineral balance (homoeostasis) and pH level within the body fluids.

In addition to being maintained at the correct volume, fluid must also be kept at the correct pH level for efficient functioning of all cells.

The body is composed of between 60 and 80 per cent water and other inorganic substances including calcium, phosphorous, potassium, magnesium, sodium, chlorine, iron and copper. Trace elements, inorganic substances found in minute quantities, include copper, iron, iodine and manganese. These substances are not found in their whole form within the body but in special combining forms known as ions. Any substance which will split into ions when dissolved in water is known as an electrolyte.

One of the most important elements in the body is hydrogen; water is a liquid compound of hydrogen and oxygen. Some substances can, when in solution, give up the hydrogen that they normally contain. These substances are known as acids. Those substances which can accept hydrogen ions are referred to as alkalis or bases.

The means of expressing the measurement of hydrogen

present in any given substance is through the pH level. This is marked on a scale of $0-14$ with 7 being neutral, a lower figure acidic and a higher figure alkaline. The average pH of body fluids is 7.4 — slightly alkaline. The pH must be maintained at a constant level to ensure correct cell function; this maintenance is referred to as homeostasis. Through selective reabsorption by the kidneys, the balance of electrolytes, and therefore the pH, within the body fluids is maintained.

5) Non-excretory functions of the kidneys are:

To produce the hormone erythropoietin, which is transported via the bloodstream to the bone marrow which it stimulates into producing more red blood cells.

To convert vitamin D into its active form.

The composition of urine

The urine of grass-kept horses is alkaline because of the salt and mineral content of grasses. Hay and short feeds may cause the urine of a stabled horse to be slightly acidic as a result of protein breakdown. A healthy horse will excrete an average of 5 litres (9 pints) every twenty-four hours. The approximate composition will be: 96 per cent water; 2 per cent urea (the by-product of protein metabolism); 2 per cent salts, some bile pigments and hormones.

In the event of infection, the urine will also contain toxins eliminated from the system by the kidneys. Although it contains large quantities of calcium carbonate crystals, the urine of a healthy horse is more or less clear and is free from offensive odour.

Discolouration of the urine may be indicative of disorders:

If dark red to near black — coloured with the muscle pigment myoglobin when azoturia has occurred.

If blood-coloured, urinary calculi may be present.

Also, if the urine is odorous, there may be infection of the bladder.

DISORDERS OF THE URINARY SYSTEM

Cystitis

Inflammation of the bladder.

Causes

May be a result of invading micro-organisms from the kidneys via the ureters or, in a mare, from an infected vagina via the urethra.

Signs

The horse may appear to be attempting to urinate without success, or repeatedly straining and producing small quantities of urine; blood and/or pus may be seen in the urine. The urine may be foul smelling. There may be a raised temperature.

Treatment

This will vary according to the cause. If bacterial, antibiotics will be used. Encourage the horse to drink freely to ensure a free flow of urine.

Cystitis may lead to pyelitis — an infection of the pelvis of the kidney, characterised by pus in the urine. Treatment of pyelitis involves the administration of antibiotics and, as with cystitis, encouraging the horse to drink.

Nephritis

Inflammation of the kidney.

Causes

A rare condition, most often seen in newborn foals, which results from an Actinobacillus spp. infection and occasionaly follows strangles. Inflammation of the kidney may also occur as a result of a blow to the loin area, for example after a fall.

Signs

May include one or a combination of the following:

Generally depressed state with a loss of appetite.

Stiffness in movement.

Rise in temperature.

Treatment
This will depend upon the cause but, where it results from bacterial infection, antibiotics may be administered.

Urinary calculi

As mentioned earlier, large quantities of calcium carbonate crystals are normal in equine urine and do not constitute a bladder problem. However, gradual deposition of salts from the urine may cause the formation of a calculus or stone in the pelvis of the kidney, bladder or urethra. Calculi may be formed from calcium carbonate, phosphates, blood proteins, blood and tissue cells.

Signs
These are similar to cystitis in clinical appearance:

There may be frequent attempts to urinate and the horse may pass blood in the urine.

Abdominal pain: the horse may walk with a stilted gait.

Upon rectal examination the bladder may feel distended — the horse may need to be tranquillized to facilitate this examination. The calculus may be felt most easily when the bladder is empty.

Treatment
If the calculus is within the urethra, the vet may administer a smooth muscle relaxant to aid the passage of the stone. If this fails, surgery will be necessary.

Very often the calculi form in the pelvis of the kidney and pass into the bladder where they increase in size. Calculi in the bladder will need to be removed surgically.

After surgery the horse must have a good supply of drinking water available. The addition of electrolytes to the water may help to promote the flow of urine.

Leptospirosis

This is a contagious disease affecting animals and man. In the horse, leptospirosis is usually a mild disease with a good prognosis. In man, it can be fatal.

Cause

It is caused by the bacteria Leptospira pomana. These microorganisms are generally water-borne and infection may occur as a result of contact with infective urine or urine-contaminated feed — rodents may infect feedstuffs. (In man, the inhalation of urinary vapours can lead to infection.) Following infection, Leptospires often accumulate in the kidneys and are shed in the urine for a long time.

Signs

Rise in temperature — 103−105 °F (39.5−40.5 °C).

Depression and dullness.

Loss of appetite and condition.

Jaundice symptoms.

Possible abortion in pregnant mares.

Inflammation of the iris, ciliary body and choroid coat of the eyeball. This condition is known as periodic opthalmia and is an intermittent recurrent disease that can lead eventually to blindness.

Treatment

The vet will administer antibiotics — penicillin is effective. The prognosis is generally good, although the disease can be fatal in foals.

Ruptured bladder in foals

The exact cause is unknown but it may be related to trauma and pressure during the birth process. It is more common in colt foals, who have a longer urethra.

Signs

The signs typically appear on the third day of life; the foal strains and develops a crouching posture and may show signs of colic. The abdomen becomes distended with free urine. Urine may be passed, but only in small quantities.

Diagnosis is confirmed by ultrasound scanning of the abdomen where abundant free fluid is seen, and sampling the peritoneal fluid which contains high quantities of the urine constituents, urea and creatinine.

Treatment

This is by surgical correction of the defect in the bladder wall. Before anaesthetizing the foal, the free urine is drained using a cannula and the acid:base and electrolyte imbalances that have developed are corrected.

8

THE SICK HORSE

So far, we have looked at diseases which relate specifically to individual parts of the body. In this chapter, we will look more globally at physiological malfunction, its causes and cures.

CAUSES OF PHYSIOLOGICAL MALFUNCTION

Physiological malfunction generally occurs as a result of one or a combination of the following:

Injury. Damage to bone and tissue can occur as a result of an accident when working, in transit or simply whilst out in the field. An injury may be further complicated by the effects of haemorrhaging (which can lead to shock) and the risk of infection. The initial injury management and subsequent recovery and rehabilitation programme will largely govern the outcome.

Nutritional imbalance. This covers a multitude of factors which may range from the provision of a poor diet lacking in vital nutrients to the ingestion of poison. The latter may cause severe malfunctioning of the major organs, in particular, the liver.

Apart from causing nutritional imbalance, provision of poor quality feedstuffs can lead to the inhalation of mould spores, resulting in an allergic reaction. Moreover, moulding feedstuffs produce fungal growths which, in turn, produce toxic substances, the ingestion of which can lead to mycotoxicosis (poisoning by fungi).

The ingestion of toxins in various forms is dealt with more fully further on (Poisoning).

Parasitic infestation. Internal parasites can cause severe damage to major organs and blood vessels. This topic has been covered fully in another book in this series, *The Horse: General Management.*

Invasion by pathogenic (disease-causing) microbes. These microbes include fungi, bacteria and viruses. The diseases caused as a result of their invasion are, to a certain extent, controlled by the horse's internal defence mechanisms, but if these are insufficient, the resources of veterinary knowledge are required. Efficient isolation procedures and good sick nursing are also vital if disease is to be controlled.

Fungal disease may be caused by the direct invasion of the tissues by fungi (for example, ringworm), or through inhalation of fungal spores found in hay and bedding, leading to obstructive pulmonary disease. However, the most common cause of infectious disease is invasion by pathogenic bacteria or viruses, and it is these causes we shall consider further.

Defining bacteria

Bacteria are the simplest single-celled micro-organisms found throughout the environment. They measure approximately 0.001 mm, and an area of $6.5 \, \text{cm}^2$ (one square inch) can accommodate approximately nine trillion bacteria. However, bacteria may be seen through a normal light microscope. It is worth mentioning that not all bacteria are harmful. Many have a positively useful function, for example the bacteria in the large intestine ferment cellulose, thus aiding its digestion.

Structure

Most bacteria have a strong, rigid cell wall made of cellulose, which provides support and protection for the protoplast within. Protoplast consists of cytoplasm containing several small structures.

These structures include ribosomes — minute granules containing ribonucleic acid (RNA) which are responsible for protein synthesis, inclusion granules (larger granules used as food reserves) and the chromatid body or nucleoid — a continuous ring of deoxyribo-nucleic acid (DNA), a single chromosome containing all of the bacterium's genes.

Bacteria do not have a nucleus. A plasma membrane just inside the cell wall controls the passage of materials in and out of the cell.

Classification

Bacteria are classified according to their shape:

Cocci —   spherical cells.

Bacilli —   cylindrical, rod-shaped cells.

Vibrios —   comma-shaped rods.

Spirilla —   spiral-shaped rods.

Clostridium —   drumstick shape.

Streptococci —   a string of spherical cells.

The name given to each type of bacteria is derived from the binominal system universally applied in biology. The first name indicates the small group of similar organisms to which it belongs — the genus. This name always has a capital letter (upper case). The second name is that of the particular species and always starts with a lower case letter (for example, Streptococcus equi).

Bacteria are also broadly classified according to their uptake of a laboratory stain: Gram negative or Gram positive — a point relative in terms of antibiotic spectrums.

Methods of feeding

Bacteria have different methods of obtaining food:

Autotrophic bacteria are self-feeding and hence free-living. Although they do not contain chlorophyll they make their own food using energy from sunlight (photosynthesis).

Saprophytic bacteria feed on dead organic matter. Enzymes from the bacteria pass through the cell wall to digest material. Once digested, the nutrients are absorbed back into the cytoplasm.

Parasitic bacteria gain nutriment from their host.

Reproduction

Bacteria usually reproduce asexually by simple binary fission; one cell divides into two, two cells divide into four and so on. Aerobic bacteria reproduce in the presence of oxygen whilst anaerobic bacteria will only reproduce in the absence of oxygen. Reproduction occurs very quickly when there is an adequate supply of nutrients combined with suitable conditions; optimum temperature, pH and oxygen levels. In such conditions one cell is capable of producing over a million more in only a few hours.

In the reproductive process, nutrients are taken into the cell and converted into nucleic acids and proteins, resulting in an increase in cell size. The cell elongates and a dividing wall known as a septum begins to form. Once this is formed, the cell divides into two.

Some bacteria are able to remain dormant when conditions are not conducive to reproduction. They produce a tough spore (endospore) contained within a thick protective wall. This endospore is resistant to drying out, heat, disinfectants etc. Clostridium tetani (the agent which causes tetanus) is an example. The endospores survive dormant in the soil, awaiting the opportunity to enter a wound and transform into growing, reproducing bacteria cells.

Bacteria and disease

Some bacteria are invariably pathogenic, that is, they always cause disease, while some only cause disease when the body's defence mechanism is weakened. The bacteria's capacity to produce disease, — its virulence — is dependent upon its ability to invade, become established and multiply within the host. Bacteria produce disease by:

Causing direct damage to the body cells.

Producing poisonous substances (toxins), the action of which causes cell breakdown and/or interference with normal cell function.

Provoking inflammation which leads to the symptoms of disease.

Causing an allergic reaction as the host forms the antibody needed to fight off the pathogenic attack.

In order to produce disease the bacteria generally have to enter the tissues of the host. Having gained entry they may remain at that site and multiply. This is known as local spread, an example of which is Streptococcus equi, which remains in the throat region and causes strangles. Systemic spread is when the bacteria spread throughout the body, often using the lymphatic and/or the blood circulatory system as a means of transportation.

Bacteria may enter the body through the skin, conjunctiva and the mucosal lining of the alimentary, respiratory and urino-genital tracts. Such entry is generally prevented by the external defence mechanisms. These include:

The skin, which offers protection until it is torn.

Tears, which wash bacteria away from the conjunctiva.

Mucous membranes; the mucus produced traps organisms. Also, the lining cells are impenetrable to most bacteria unless they are damaged by the bacteria themselves or by lack of blood flow (as in twisted gut).

The cilia. Within the respiratory tract, hairlike cilia 'sweep' mucus and bacteria away from the lungs.

Coughing, sweating, urinating and defecating help to flush unwanted bacteria out of the body.

Lactic acid and fatty acids help maintain a low pH which inhibits harmful bacteria.

The normal bacterial flora in the gut compete for nutrients and produce inhibitory substances.

When bacteria pass these external defences, the body's resistance to pathogenic invasion is dependent upon the efficiency of the internal defence mechanisms.

Internal defences against bacteria

These are:

Inflammation

As a result of bacterial activity, toxins are produced and cells damaged. This causes capillaries and lymphatic vessels to dilate and become more permeable, a reaction which is manifest as inflammation. Cells such as phagocytes, together with antibodies (see below) are attracted to the area and pass more easily from the blood to the affected site.

Phagocytosis

Phagocytosis literally means 'cell eating'. Neutrophils, the white blood cells otherwise known as polymorphs, circulate in the blood and are the most active type of phagocyte.

Another type of white blood cell, monocytes, originate in the lymphatic system and are situated at all lymph nodes ready to destroy organisms by phagocytosis. Macrophages (monocytes which have moved into the tissues and increased in size) in the lungs and spleen, also combat bacteria and viruses which enter cells.

There are two stages of phagocytosis:

1) Attachment — the phagocyte attaches itself to the bacterium or foreign protein. This is easier if the bacterium has a small capsule and is covered in antibody.

2) Ingestion — the bacterium is enclosed and killed. The neutrophil produces various enzymes which breaks down the bacterium.

Some bacteria are very resistant to ingestion and may actually kill the phagocyte. A large number of dead neutrophils will cause the formation of pus.

Bacteriacidal substances

Many body secretions contain substances which inhibit or destroy bacteria, for example acid in the stomach kills ingested organisms. Non-pathogenic bacteria are always present in the large intestine and are prevented from being absorbed by the mucous membrane defence mechanism.

Within the serum is a complex system of proteins known as complement, which is the body's main bacteriacidal substance. It assists antibodies in the destruction of bacteria. When antibodies attach themselves to pathogenic bacteria complement recognizes this and produces more of its own molecules to assist. It also produces an enzyme which breaks down the bacterial cells as well as encouraging inflammation and phagocytosis.

Toxins and antibody production

Toxins are poisonous substances and may be broadly split into two categories; exotoxins and endotoxins.

Exotoxins are very powerful soluble protein poisons, produced and secreted by living bacterial cells. The presence of such a toxin represents an antigen. An antigen is a foreign substance that stimulates the production of a specific antibody. The antibody to a toxin is known as an antitoxin. Antibodies are proteins formed by the plasma cells of the lymphatic system in response to the presence of an antigen. They have the following effects:

They make phagocytosis easier by attaching to the antibody.

They stop bacteria from attaching to mucosal surfaces.

They neutralize toxins.

They activate the production of complement which stimulates inflammation and increases the supply of phagocytes.

The production of antibodies can be stimulated by introducing small doses of the relevant exotoxin into the body. This is done so that the antitoxin which is produced may be separated from the blood and stored ready for use in the treatment of an affected animal. A specific exotoxin can be treated in the laboratory to produce a non-poisonous substance known as toxoid. When injected into the body, toxoid stimulates the production of antitoxin which provides immunity from the pathogenic effects of that toxin, should it ever reappear in the horse's system. For example, tetanus toxoid is used to provide immunity against tetanus. This topic is discussed further under Vaccination.

Endotoxins are produced within certain bacteria and dispensed only upon the death of the micro-organism. Specific antitoxins are available for a few of the endotoxins. Antiendotoxic drugs (such as flunixin) stabilize endothelial linings of blood vessels to prevent shock produced by increased vascular permeability.

Defining viruses

Viruses are smaller than bacteria; it is only possible to see them through an electron microscope. They consist of a simple protein sheath around either a DNA or RNA strand. DNA (deoxyribonucleic acid) and RNA (ribonucleic acid) are substances concerned with the storage of genetic information. Most viruses are pathogenic and can be transmitted from one animal to another quite easily. Viruses are always parasitic − they are only able to multiply using the enzymes of the host's cells, which results in the death of those cells. They reproduce by replication. Viral nucleic acid (either DNA or RNA) is either injected into the host cell or the virus enters the host cell and 'directs' it to manufacture more virus cells.

Viruses cannot be controlled with antibiotics.

Major differences between bacteria and viruses

The differences can be summarized thus:

BACTERIA	VIRUSES
Larger.	Smaller.
Has cell wall.	No cell wall.
Produces own enzymes for metabolism and reproduction.	Depends upon the host cell's enzymes.
Usually reproduces by binary fission.	Never reproduces by binary fission.
Contains both DNA and RNA.	Contains either, never both.
Can multiply outside host cells.	Only multiplies within living cells.
Some form toxins.	None form toxins.
Can be sacrophytic or parasitic.	Always parasitic.

Vaccination

Vaccination is the method of producing active immunity against a specific viral or bacterial infection by inoculating with a vaccine. A vaccine is the preparation containing the necessary antigen, which may be viral or bacterial. Once specific antibodies have been produced, defence against that disease is established, that is to say the horse is actively immune and will therefore have his own internal defence mechanism against that particular disease.

Passive immunity is a more short-lived protection offered by the small amounts of antibodies passed from the mare to her foal via the placenta and/or the colostrum.

There are two main types of vaccine:

Killed vaccine (dead or inactivated). The antigenic preparation is derived from dead micro-organisms. Some are made more effective through the addition of adjuvants. These are substances which, by slowing down the rate of release of the antigen from the vaccine, enhance the immune response. Vaccines to which adjuvants have been added are known as adjuvenated vaccines. Greater amounts of antibodies are produced when encountering an antigen for the second time. For this reason, two injections given fairly close together may be needed at the onset of a vaccination programme.

The protection afforded by such vaccines is short-term, for example the drug used to prevent widespread viral abortion on studs (Pneumabort K) has to be administered every two months.

Live vaccine. Living organisms are weakened (attenuated) so they will not cause the disease. Generally, these vaccines are very potent and immunity will last longer once the primary course has been given (for example tetanus vaccine is effective for eighteen to twenty-four months).

DRUGS

Any chemical compound that can be administered to the horse and cause a change within the body may be described as a drug. These compounds have many uses and may be divided into groups according to their actions and effects. The administration of drugs to influence the performance of a competition horse is known as doping, an activity which is illegal among the governing equestrian bodies such as the Jockey Club, FEI and BSJA. All drugs should be administered under the instruction of a vet and the instructions regarding the amount and frequency of dosing followed. There are often side effects to consider and misuse of any drug may prove harmful to the horse, especially as individual horses may respond differently to certain drugs.

Drugs may be broadly divided into two groups: those to restore normal performance and those which alter normal behaviour or performance.

Drugs to restore normal performance

Included in this group are:

Anti-inflammatories and analgesics.

Antibiotics.

Bronchodilators.

Diuretics.

Anti-inflammatories and analgesics (pain relievers)

These may be broadly divided into two main groups; steroidal and non-steroidal. The chief steroidal anti-inflammatories are the corticosteroids.

Corticosteroids

Steroids are chemical substances made up of fatty acids which may be derived from both plant and animal tissue. Cholesterol is the major steroid in the body and is chemically linked to some digestive acids and hormones. The hormones produced by the adrenal cortex (the outer layer of the adrenal gland: *ad*; near to, *renal*; kidneys) have a common basic biochemical structure and are called steroids. These hormones may be arranged into three groups:

Adrenal sex hormones.

Mineralocorticoids.

Glucocorticoids.

The latter two groups are referred to as corticosteroids.

Mineralocorticoids include hormones such as aldosterone, which helps to regulate electrolyte levels within the extracellular fluids by promoting excretion of potassium and retention of sodium.

The release of glucocorticoids is controlled by adrenocortico-trophic hormone (ACTH) produced by the anterior pituitary gland. The two main compounds, cortisol and corticosterone, are responsible for raising blood sugar levels, increasing glycogen storage in the liver and have anti-inflammatory properties.

They do, however, cause the body to retain sodium and water.

Synthetic corticosteroids are now widely used as drugs because they cause less sodium retention than the natural compound, cortisol, which was used originally. However, when large amounts of artificial corticosteroids are present the amount of ACTH released from the anterior pituitary gland is reduced. ACTH is normally released when the horse needs more natural corticosteroid in times of stress, injury etc.

It is not known exactly how corticosteroids reduce inflammation but, in addition to reducing the bad effects, they also reduce the good by lowering the level of antibodies at the site of the inflammation, which leaves the area more prone to infection. This point must be carefully considered when injecting a corticosteroid directly into a joint, for example when treating an arthritic condition.

At therapeutic dosages, corticosteroids produce the following effects:

1) They depress lymphoid tissue activity.

2) They stabilize the packages of destructive enzymes within phagocytes.

3) They reduce capillary permeability.

4) They reduce neutrophil recruitment.

They are not normally used in infectious conditions as they reduce the body's ability to fight infection.

Non-steroidal anti-inflammatory drugs (NSAIDs)
These drugs have similar effects to corticosteroids but are chemically unrelated to them. NSAIDs are acidic chemicals which accumulate in areas of inflammation. They have a less wide-ranging anti-inflammatory action than corticosteroids and do not incapacitate the ability to fight infection. Their actions are:

1) Antipyretic (reduce fever).

2) Anti-inflammatory.

3) Analgesic.

A group of substances which exert similar effects to those of hormones occur in many body tissues. These substances, prostaglandins, are responsible for the symptoms of inflammation in areas of injury or infection. Prostaglandins form as a result of the action of a catalystic enzyme, cyclooxygenase, on the fatty acid, arachidonic acid.

NSAIDs reduce inflammation by neutralizing the cyclo-oxygenase. The drugs are broken down in the liver into inactive substances known as metabolites, which are then eliminated via the bile or urine. The presence of these metabolites may be detected in urine for a much longer period than in the blood and at higher concentrations.

The longest established and most commonly used NSAID is phenylbutazone ('bute'), which may be administered orally as paste or granules or injected intravenously. Phenylbutazone is absorbed in the small intestine — if administered before the horse has eaten, more of the drug will be absorbed. The acidic nature of bute can lead to interference with the mucous secretions in the stomach and ulceration within the intestines and, occasionally, of the tongue. This problem may occur if it is used over a prolonged period, especially in small ponies or horses showing a sensitive reaction to the drug. When bute is broken down in the liver, a small proportion breaks down into a clinically active metabolite called oxyphenbutazone.

Bute is very effective in the treatment of bony disorders such as arthritis, but less effective on muscular inflammation such as that incurred with azoturia. In this condition a newer, more expensive drug called naproxen is often used. Naproxen has a very low toxicity and is broken down quickly within the body. In order to maintain effective levels, this drug has to be administered twice daily.

Other types of NSAID which may be prescribed by the vet include meclofenamic acid and flunixin. Meclofenamic acid is very potent; it is estimated to be twelve times more effective than bute. However, levels need to be built up — the effects may be seen from thirty-six to ninety-six hours after dosage. Administration is always oral.

Flunixin, the newest of the NSAIDs, may be administered orally or injected intravenously or intramuscularly. It has proved to be a very effective analgesic when treating colic. It is, however, important to stress that flunixin must only be used in colic when a specific diagnosis has been made. It is a very effective anti-endotoxic and will mask the signs of deterioration (twisted gut) so that it becomes too late to save the patient with surgery. It could, therefore, be lethal for an owner to give flunixin (trade name Finadyne) to a horse with colic before a vet has made sure that a surgical lesion is not present.

The BSJA, FEI and Jockey Club publish, in their current rule books, lists of forbidden substances which must not be administered to either horse or rider prior to a competition. Tests for these may be carried out at any time during the course of a competition. The BSJA does not, at present, include phenylbutazone and its metabolite, oxyphenbutazone, on its list. Under FEI rules these two drugs were tested for on a quantitative basis but, as of 1994, the FEI has banned bute completely. This ruling has been the subject of much debate. If it is necessary to administer bute to a competition horse for any reason, veterinary advice must be sought to ensure that no trace of the drug is present in the bloodstream or urine at the time of competition.

Antibiotics

Antibiotics are chemical compounds derived from living organisms which are either bactericidal (kill bacteria) or bacteriostatic (inhibit bacterial reproduction). Antibiotics may act in one or more of the following ways:

By breaking down the bacterial cell wall.

By affecting the cell membrane.

By interfering with protein synthesis and therefore inhibiting reproduction, possibly causing death of the cell.

Antibiotics may be classified as narrow- or broad-spectrum according to the range of bacteria against which they are effective. Types of antibiotic include:

Penicillin. This is the best known antibiotic, being the first ever to be discovered and used. Penicillin is a narrow-spectrum (for Gram-positive bacteria only) bactericidal compound which acts on the cell walls. Following an injection, penicillin is readily absorbed and diffused into the bloodstream.

It is non-toxic even in very large doses. Semi-synthetic penicillins have been developed to overcome the disadvantages of the narrow-spectrum factor. Penicillin may be used in the treatment of strangles (Streptococcus equi), wounds and the prevention of sepsis during surgery.

Sulphonamides. These complex synthetic compounds are bacteriostatic to susceptible organisms, for example Streptococci. There are several types in veterinary use, the most popular being sulphanilamide, which is used extensively as a dry dressing for wounds. Sulphonamides are widely used in combination with trimethoprim.

Streptomycin. This is a narrow-spectrum bactericidal compound which affects protein synthesis within the bacterial cell.

Tetracyclines. These are broad-spectrum bacteriostatic antibiotics, which work by interfering with protein synthesis within the bacterial cell. They must be administered with great care; they can cause a disturbance of the gut flora, resulting in varying levels of potentially fatal diarrhoea. Tetracyclines can cause irritation and are not suitable for use in very young stock or pregnant mares.

Bronchodilators

These are drugs which act upon the respiratory system. Their functions have been discussed earlier under the treatment of respiratory diseases.

Diuretics

These drugs reduce blood pressure and cause diuresis — the copious excretion of urine. The kidneys are encouraged to excrete large quantities of sodium and, therefore, water. The most commonly used diuretic is frusemide, marketed as Lasix. This is widely used in America for racehorses as a means of preventing exercise-induced pulmonary haemorrhage (EIPH), which is thought to be caused as a result of high blood pressure in the pulmonary capillaries. The use of a diuretic is thought to ease the pulmonary oedema by eliminating fluids from the body.

Drugs to alter normal behaviour or performance

Included in this group are:

Stimulants.

Depressants.

Anabolic steroids.

The main function of the central nervous system (CNS) is to co-ordinate the responses of the various organs of the body by providing the chief communication network. Therefore any compound which affects the CNS will cause far-reaching reactions throughout the body. Messages are transmitted between nerve cells by means of neurotransmitter substances which pass from one cell to another. Certain drugs can influence the production of these neurotransmitter substances; stimulants will accelerate production while depressants inhibit production.

Stimulants

Given prior to a competition, these increase the response of the CNS. The most common drugs in this group may be subdivided again, into amphetamines, xanthines and narcotics.

Amphetamines. These compounds cause the same physiological responses in the body as adrenalin, the hormone responsible for increased cardiac and respiratory output, which leads to stronger blood flow to the muscles and improved oxygen uptake. Glucose and free fatty acids are released to provide extra energy to the muscles.

Xanthines. These include caffeine, a compound of which is theobromine. This substance is found in some plants and therefore may be found in certain pelleted feeds. Feed manufacturers have to ensure that their products are free from theobromine if they are to meet the Jockey Club requirements.

Narcotics. These are morphine-related drugs. Morphine is one of the chief derivatives of the poppy. When used in man, it produces analgesia and narcosis. However, when a morphine-related drug is used in the horse, a state of acute stimulation is induced. Morphine and its related compounds exert their effects by acting on specific receptors within the CNS. The body produces natural morphine-like substances known as endorphins, which have an analgesic effect. The use of the twitch on the muzzle is thought to cause endorphins to be released into the system. Unlike morphine-related drugs, they have a calming effect.

Depressants

The horse can be made less responsive to his surroundings through the administration of drugs which slow down the passage of nervous impulses within the CNS. Such drugs include tranquillizers, sedatives and B-adrenergic blocking agents. The subject of tranquillizers and sedatives is discussed in another book in this series, *The Horse: General Management.* The most commonly used sedative is Acepromazine, otherwise known as ACP.

B-adrenergic blocking agents are drugs which inhibit the normal metabolic and physiological responses to exercise by blocking the actions of adrenalin. This results in a greatly reduced capacity to perform.

Anabolic steroids

Anabolic steroids are compounds synthesised with chemical structures derived from testosterone, which promote the building of tissue (anabolism). This leads to increased muscle mass, which may improve performance and delay the onset of fatigue. The muscular appearance of a horse may also be improved artificially prior to sale.

The most commonly used anabolic steroid is nandrolene. However, use of these compounds in horses is forbidden.

FURTHER CAUSES OF SICKNESS IN THE HORSE

Poisoning

A poison is a substance either formed in or taken into the body which impairs the healthy functioning of the cells, possibly resulting in death. Poisons are usually ingested but may be inhaled or taken in through the skin. As previously mentioned, some bacteria produce harmful toxins, but many useful medicines and minerals can, in large doses, be poisonous – for example an overdose of anthelmintic (wormer) can be harmful.

Poisoning can take several forms and may affect the central nervous system. The horse may show a combination of the following signs:

He may become very lethargic, hanging his head low or resting it on a convenient object.

He may walk around in circles and show signs of inco-ordination.

Diarrhoea.

Colic.

Dilation or constriction of the pupils.

Distressed breathing.

Blood in the urine.

Jaundice.

Convulsions, coma, death.

If ever poisoning is suspected the vet must be called immediately. Poisoning may be suspected whenever a horse falls ill suddenly after a change of feed type or pasture. As preventative measures, paddocks should be checked to ensure that no hedge or shrub cuttings are thrown over the fence. Fallen acorns must be raked up and removed. Hay should be checked for contamination by foxgloves or ragwort. Also, note that many plants produce powerful toxins. Further information on this topic is available on another book in this series, *The Horse: General Management*.

Jaundice and diarrhoea, major signs of poisoning, are worthy of further explanation.

Jaundice

In many cases, toxins are absorbed from the stomach and gut by the bloodstream — the more soluble the poison, the faster this absorption will occur. Once absorbed, the toxins are transported to the largest gland in the body, the liver. The liver plays a very important role in the excretion of toxic products which enter the body through, or are produced in, the gut. Poisons are broken down here, along with exhausted red blood cells which are changed into bile pigments. Bile, synthesised in the liver and secreted into the duodenum, aids the absorption of fats. It is a greenish-yellow fluid which, being alkaline, neutralizes the acid chyme which passes from the stomach and enters the duodenum as part of the digestive process. Bile pigments are excreted from the body in the faeces and urine. If excretion is slower than absorption, toxic substances will accumulate in the body. These poisons attack the liver and hinder the breakdown of bile, resulting in an accumulation of bile pigments in the blood. The build-up of bile pigments causes a yellowing of the membranes, known as jaundice. The urine may also be very dark; a brownish-yellow in colour.

Jaundice can also be caused in other ways, such as blockage of the bile ducts by tumours, parasites or inflammation. Excessive destruction of red blood cells leads to the overproduction of bile pigments, results in the yellowing of the membranes. Other contributing conditions include anaemia and haemolytic disease.

Treatment involves removing the cause, that is to say determining the poison and, if possible, administering the antidote. An antidote is an agent which counteracts the poison by preventing or arresting its harmful effects.

Diarrhoea

Diarrhoea is not an actual disease but an indication that something is wrong. Some cases of diarrhoea improve without specific treatment. However, prolonged diarrhoea impairs the absorption of nutrients and other digestive processes and, most importantly, leads to dehydration which, if untreated, can be fatal. Therefore, if the diarrhoea is very severe and/or the horse has not recovered within forty-eight hours, the vet should be called.

Causes

Feeding contaminated, mouldy feedstuffs.

Altering the diet suddenly.

Feedstuffs intended for another type of animal, for example pig nuts instead of Horse and Pony cubes.

Worm infestation.

Salmonellosis.

Colitis X.

Reaction to antibiotic therapy.

Stress/excitement.

Poisoning.

The vet will examine the horse noting:

Temperature.

Pulse.

Body condition — weight loss and dehydration.

Condition of teeth — is the horse able to chew his food properly?

Gut movements.

Faeces — volume, consistency, presence of blood.

Diagnosis is aided by blood tests and bacteriological culture of the faeces.

Specific causes of poisoning

While there are many substances which are potentially toxic to horses, the following are examples of some common causes which should be guarded against:

Toxins produced by micro-organisms

Botulism

Botulism had not been frequently reported until big bale silage started to be used as fodder for horses.

This condition is caused by the toxins of the bacteria Clostridium botulinum which is present in the soil and is a fairly common contaminant of animal feedstuffs. Well made silage must reach a pH level of 4.5 as quickly as possible and contain at least 25 per cent dry matter to prevent the growth of harmful bacteria. Once the contaminated silage has been ingested, signs may show within three to seven days depending upon the quantities eaten.

Signs include general weakness, difficulty in eating and progressive paralysis which results in the horse moving with a shuffling, stiff gait, dragging the toes along the ground. He may stand with his head and neck distended. Respiratory paralysis may occur, resulting in death.

Diagnosis is generally made upon examination of the feedstuffs. The vet may administer food, liquid paraffin and electrolytes via a stomach tube — this has proved helpful in the small percentage of cases who have survived.

Prevention of botulism involves never feeding contaminated/spoiled feedstuffs and only using big bale silage if the bag is intact, the pH level is 4.0–4.5 and there is a good aroma and no sign of moulds.

It is possible to provide immunity through vaccination.

Mycotoxicosis (poisoning by fungi)

All feedstuffs, especially those with a high moisture content, are susceptible to moulding. Feedstuffs may sometimes become contaminated either before or after the harvesting stages of feed production. These should not be fed to horses.

Fungal growths produce toxic metabolites known as myco-toxins — the effect produced by these toxins is known as mycotoxicosis.

Poisoning may be shown as colicky pain or, in more severe cases, as neurological disorder.

Salmonellosis

There are over 1,000 different types of bacteria in the salmonella group of which some forty may affect horses. The disease causes serious illness in youngstock and generally affects horses in a debilitated, stressed state. Occasionally there may be an outbreak as a result of a contaminated food or water supply.

Causes

The primary source of infection may be from a contaminated water supply — salmonella organisms may be present in domestic sewage which pollutes streams. Alternatively, animal feeds and farm slurry may be contaminated. The organism tends to thrive in the large intestine and associated lymph nodes. The bacteria which most commonly affects horses is Salmonella typhimurium.

Carrier horses are generally asymptomatic (they show no symptoms) but they can pass the disease on by shedding the organisms either continually or intermittently in their droppings.

Signs

Salmonellosis generally occurs in four forms:

Peracute. This form mainly affects foals. The symptoms, which arise suddenly, are:

Temperature rise to 104−106 °F (40−41 °C).

Depression and weakness.

Loss of appetite.

Increased heart rate and weak pulse.

Increased respiratory rate.

Blueing of mucous membranes.

Abdominal pain and diarrhoea, with latter leading to dehydration and electrolyte imbalance.

Death usually occurs within approximately seventy-two hours.

Acute. This form mainly affects adult equines. The symptoms, again sudden, are:

Temperature rise to 104–106 °F (40–41 °C).

Depression and weakness.

Loss of appetite.

Increased heart rate and weakened pulse.

Increased respiratory rate.

Diarrhoea — this sometimes does not develop for a few days but then leads to dehydration and electrolyte imbalance.

Some horses survive, and of those that do some:

1) recover fully and are not carriers.

2) become asymptomatic carriers but never shed the organisms.

3) become asymptomatic carriers and shed intermittently or continually.

4) become chronic cases.

Chronic. Signs which may continue in survivors of the acute form include:

Often, damage to the intestinal lining.

Loss of condition.

Possible loss of appetite.

Soft faeces and intermittent diarrhoea.

The horse may eventually die or need to be destroyed.

Atypical. This may occur after a stressful situation such as transportation, competition or undergoing surgery.

High temperature; 103−106 °F (39.5−41 °C).

Loss of appetite.

Depression.

Mild abdominal pain.

Soft faeces.

The horse generally recovers within a few days.

Treatment
The vet will confirm the diagnosis of salmonellosis through the results of faecal culture.

Fluid and electrolyte therapy is essential to combat dehydration.

Plasma, blood or plasma volume expander therapy may be needed.

The vet may use antibiotics.

It is of great importance that the horse is isolated and that the rules of isolation are strictly adhered to.

It should be noted that *there is a risk of this disease being transmitted to humans,* so precautions must be taken to ensure that it is not passed on to those in contact with the sick horse. These precautions include the use of overalls and rubber gloves, and extreme attention to hygiene − arm and hand scrubbing, etc.

Toxins from other sources

Anticoagulants

Poisoning may occur as a result of an overdose of a chemical substance such as Warfarin used therapeutically, for example in the treatment of navicular syndrome, or through eating anticoagulant rodenticides.

Signs may include external bleeding that will not clot, internal bleeding, colic if the abdomen is affected, pale mucous membranes and swellings beneath the skin, particularly over the joints.

The vet will administer vitamin K to promote synthesis of the blood-clotting agents.

Cyanide poisoning

Cyanide may be used in fumigants, fertilizers and rodenticides. Furthermore, certain plants contain cyanogenetic compounds which, in response to the actions of enzymes during digestion, yield hydrocyanic (prussic) acid. Examples of such plants include arrow grass, wild black cherry, choke cherry and flax.

Linseed is the seed of the flax plant and must, for the reasons given, be soaked overnight before being boiled for at least ten minutes to destroy the prussic acid. The seeds are then simmered until jellified.

Signs of cyanide/prussic acid poisoning include salivation, increase in the respiratory rate, muscle tremors and spasms. The horse may struggle and stagger about before collapsing and dying. Therefore, as soon as poisoning is suspected, the vet must be called.

Lead poisoning

This may be caused through ingesting vegetation contaminated by mining operations, or through chewing woodwork painted with lead paints. Accidental contamination of feedstuffs will lead to an outbreak of lead poisoning.

Signs include a loss of appetite, weight loss, depression, muscular weakness, joint stiffness, colic, diarrhoea and anaemia. Sometimes laryngeal paralysis will occur, which may result in pneumonia.

Selenium poisoning

Selenium is a vital trace element within the horse's diet but, if eaten in large quantities, it is highly toxic. Plants or grains containing high levels of selenium tend to grow in areas of very low rainfall. The plants which accumulate selenium may break down and degenerate into the soil. Any non-seliniferous plants which grow there subsequently may absorb the selenium and become toxic.

Signs of selenium poisoning include loss of the mane and tail, cracking of the hoof at the coronary band, general loss of condition, joint stiffness and lameness. Upon the onset of the first symptoms, call the vet and organize a soil and herbage analysis.

EQUINE VIRAL ARTERITIS (EVA)

This highly infectious viral disease had never been seen in Great Britain until the Spring of 1993, when an outbreak originated from an infected Polish stallion who had been imported in September 1992. At the time of writing the UK has no power to blanket test all imported horses or to impose import restrictions, as this would contravene EC ruling. The Ministry of Agriculture can only carry out random checks on imported animals, a factor which may contribute to further outbreaks of the disease.

EVA is transmitted via droplet infection from the nose and mouth of infected animals and via the semen of stallions who have become 'carriers' following infection.

Signs
Over 50 per cent of pregnant mares will abort, without necessarily showing other clinical signs. Otherwise:

High temperature — 105 °F (40.5 °C) for one to five days.

Loss of appetite.

Depression.

Conjunctivitis (known as 'pink eye').

Nasal discharge and congestion.

Swollen glands in the throat region.

Oedema on head and legs.

Some horses experience diarrhoea.

In foals, other signs include respiratory distress, pneumonia and colic, while mares may develop swelling of the mammary glands, and stallions swelling of the scrotum. Death may occur.

Treatment

Beyond supportive therapy treating the signs there had, until recently, been no specific treatment. A vaccine has now been developed, but it will produce a lifelong antibody which may render valuable bloodstock non-exportable under current export regulations.

Although horses who survive an attack require a long period of rest and rehabilitation, the aftermath of the disease varies between the sexes. Of those stallions who recover, about a third become carriers of the disease (known as 'shedders'). Long term shedders pass the virus on through semen only, but this renders them unusable for stud work. Infected mares recover from the worst symptoms relatively quickly and stop shedding after some three weeks, at which stage they have developed natural immunity.

NOTIFIABLE DISEASES

Under the Animal Health Act 1981 it is required that either the local Divisional Veterinary Officer of the Ministry of Agriculture or the Police are notified as soon as there is suspicion of an outbreak of any of the following diseases:

African horse sickness

This viral infection is enzootic (permanently present) in Africa. Outbreaks have occurred in the Middle East and southern Europe — in the late 1980s the disease reached Spain. The disease is prevalent in summer and autumn and is spread by biting insects which are suspected of living in another host animal, probably the dog, during the insect's inactive season.

There are three distinct clinical forms of the disease, having an incubation period which is usually five to seven days, but which may be as long as three weeks. All forms have fever symptoms, with temperature rising to 105−106 °F (40.5−41 °C). The disease has a 90 per cent mortality rate in horses and a 50 per cent mortality rate in mules and donkeys. Survivors are usually permanently debilitated.

Pulmonary Form. This acute form of the disease is the worst. With the fever sweating will be severe. The horse may collapse and die within a few hours. Respiratory distress includes coughing, frothy yellow nasal discharge and breathing difficulties. The appetite tends to be normal until the breathing difficulties prevent the horse from eating.

A very small percentage of horses do recover but have severe breathing problems for several weeks afterwards.

Cardiac Form. This is the subacute form. Signs are; colic and restlessness; cyanosis (blueing) of membranes; oedema (fluid accumulation) beneath the skin of the head, neck and chest; disturbances of the heart which include inflammation and oedema.

It may take approximately two weeks before death occurs, although a slightly larger percentage of equines recover from this form. A very long convalescence period is needed.

Third form, known as horsesickness fever. With this form the temperature rises to 105 °F (40.5 °C) within one to three days before returning to normal after three days. The horse loses appetite and condition and may exhibit slight conjunctivitis and breathing difficulties.

Laboratory diagnosis is needed to back up the clinical diagnosis in order to identify the specific strain.

Control of the disease
A vaccine is available but only offers protection against a limited number of strains. Other than this there is no treatment available except that given to alleviate the signs, therefore control of the disease is vitally important. Horses should not be kept in areas where the carrier insects are active. Repellents should be used and the horses stabled at night.

Anthrax

This acute and rapidly fatal disease occurs in all parts of the world, but especially in tropical and sub-tropical areas, where large numbers of sheep and cattle are affected each year. In the majority of other areas outbreaks are sporadic and, as a result of stringent control procedures, fairly infrequent. All animals can be affected and the disease may easily be passed on to humans.

Cause

The disease is caused by Bacillus anthracis, the spores of which are the hardest of all bacterial life to destroy. They are able to resist drying for at least two years and, if in the soil, may remain infective for at least ten years. The spores are able to resist thirty minutes boiling and are only killed with the strongest disinfectants.

Signs

Acute form. Fever; the temperature rises to 107°F (41.6°C). The central nervous system is affected, resulting in very excitable behaviour followed by depression and respiratory distress. Convulsions are then followed by coma and death occurs within forty-eight hours.

Subacute form. With this form there is colic.

The enlarged spleen may be felt by the vet upon rectal palpation.

Other signs are haemorrhaging of the mucous membranes, muscle spasm and lameness, gross swellings on the neck and lower abdomen and breathing difficulties. Death occurs within around eight days.

Chronic form. This form produces swellings on the throat, lesions on the tongue and throat and bloodstained discharge from the mouth and nose. Death is from suffocation.

Treatment

If anthrax is suspected, blood samples are not generally taken. The condition is not usually treated, because of the extreme risk of contracting the disease from the contaminated samples.

Dourine

This is a venereal disease of horses, donkeys and mules caused by Trypanosoma equiperdum, a small, single-celled parasite found in the bloodstream. It is enzootic to Africa, Asia, South America, southeast and eastern Europe. Transmission occurs during coitus. Very often the carrier animal shows no clinical signs of the disease.

Signs
The incubation period varies from two to twelve weeks. It is followed by:

Fever.

Loss of appetite.

Swelling, oedema and discharge of the genitals.

Stiffness followed by weakness and paralysis.

Extreme loss of condition.

Treatment
The vet may examine blood, oedema fluid or genital washings directly for the presence of the parasite or, alternatively, culture procedures may be used to give a definite diagnosis. Drugs effective against Trypanosomes (Trypanocidal drugs), are used.

The disease must be controlled by identification of the carrier animal and ensuring that no animals are exported from an area where the disease is enzootic.

Equine encephalomyelitis

This is a viral disease, of which there are several types, seen mainly in North and South America, Russia and the far and middle East. The viruses are insect-borne, varying in virulence but all producing the same clinical signs.

Signs
Fever.

Loss of appetite and condition.

Depression.

Drowsiness followed by violent excitability.

Collapse followed by death.

Diagnosis may prove difficult, laboratory confirmation being necessary to identify the strain of virus. The symptoms may be confused with rabies, botulism, leptospirosis or African horse sickness.

The mortality rates vary between strains, the most dangerous strain, with 90 per cent mortality, may be passed on to man.

Treatment
Fluid and electrolyte therapy.

Lowering the fever — NSAIDs are generally effective.

Protecting the horse from injury by providing a good, deep bed.

Control
Control is by annual vaccination. It is also helpful to stable horses at night and use repellents to deter insects.

Epizootic lymphangitis

This highly contagious disease spreads rapidly as a result of the fungus Histoplasma farciminosum gaining entry into the body via a skin wound or the mucous membranes. It occurs in East and West Equatorial Africa, Sudan, South Africa and parts of Asia. It is spread through either direct contact or contact with infective discharges, tools, grooming kit and equipment and also by flies.

Signs
The incubation period may be two to three months.

Lesions form on the mucous membranes of the eyes, mouth, nostrils and genitalia. A general thickening occurs along the lymphatic vessels. The lymph nodes can develop large abscesses which discharge after rupturing. Abseses and nodules which appear on the skin of the head, neck, shoulders and limbs discharge a thick, yellow pus.

These signs are, in some respects, similar signs to glanders and ulcerative lymphangitis. However, laboratory examination of a smear taken from an unopened abscess will show yeastlike cells.

The disease lasts from three to twelve months, leading to a severe loss of condition and function.

Treatment

The mortality rate is 10–15 per cent. Severe cases should be destroyed as early as possible as a means of preventing the disease from spreading. In order to control the spread, all infected horses must be isolated and any paddocks used by infected animals must not be reused for at least six months.

The only currently effective treatment is for the abscesses to be cleaned and treated with the appropriate iodide preparations.

Equine infectious anaemia

This highly contagious disease is caused by a very resistant virus, capable of remaining viable in the blood for many years. It is enzootic to the western states of America, the north-western states of Canada, Europe, Asia and Africa.

The first case in Britain was reported in 1975. Since then the disease has not often been seen in Britain.

The virus is transmitted via biting insects such as horseflies and mosquitoes, contaminated syringes and needles, or through contact with infective urine, faeces, saliva, nasal discharge, semen or milk.

Signs

Acute form. Fever – temperature rises to 105 °F (40.5 °C) and tends to fluctuate. There is also anaemia, weight loss, depression and weakness.

Subacute form. Fever for one to seven days. The temperature intermittently returns to normal. There is loss of appetite, weight loss, depression and jaundice.

Chronic form Following the weight loss typical of the other forms, some condition may be regained and the horse appears to be 'normal'. However, the symptoms may recur at any time. The virus is still present in the blood, tests upon which will also show anaemia.

Treatment
There is no specific treatment other than supportive therapy to treat the symptoms. Blood transfusions may prove beneficial.

The mortality rate varies between 30 and 70 per cent. In the acute form, death may occur in ten to thirty days. Horses in the subacute stage may die in two to three months.

Control of the disease
1) Horses should not be moved from enzootic areas. Animals to be imported from any countries known to have the disease must be blood sampled for to a specific test known as Coggins' Test.

2) The number of insect carriers should be reduced with insecticides and repellents.

3) All syringes and needles must be sterile.

4) Any animal suspected of infection must be isolated for at least forty-five and preferably ninety days.

Glanders

This is the oldest known disease of the horse, being first recorded by Hippocrates in 450 BC. It has been seen all over the world — in 1904 there were nearly 3,000 cases in Great Britain. There has been none since 1926. However, the disease is still endemic in Asia, East Africa and South America, affecting horses, donkeys, asses and mules and it is easily transmitted to man.

Causes
Glanders is caused by a bacillus, Malleomyces mallei, which may be spread through the ingestion of food and water or, less commonly, through inhalation or skin infections. It occurs in three main forms — acute and chronic respiratory, and cutaneous form. The incubation period may be several months, during which time the infected animal may be spreading the

disease to otherwise healthy animals.

Signs
Acute respiratory form (mainly seen in mules and asses).

High fever.

Ulcerations of the nasal mucous membranes with nasal discharge.

Bronchopneumonia with cough.

Nodules on lower limbs and abdomen.

Rapid loss of condition.

Death in approximately two to three weeks.

Chronic respiratory form (mainly seen in horses).

Ulceration of the passages of the upper airways with purulent nasal discharge.

Chronic pneumonia.

These symptoms may last for months.

Cutaneous form (sometimes referred to as farcy).

Nodules which appear over the body eviscerate, soften and burst, releasing a dark-coloured pus.

The lymph nodes may be enlarged and one or both of the hind limbs may become swollen.

Laboratory confirmation is needed to ensure that correct diagnosis is made. The signs may be confused with those of epizootic and ulcerative lymphangitis, pneumonia, strangles, infected tooth, guttural pouch infections or sinusitis.

Treatment
Sulphonamides are generally effective. It is, however, the policy of most countries to destroy severely affected animals as a means of aiding control of the disease. Other methods of control involve the quarantine of all infected premises and carrying out a special test known as the Mallein Test to detect

carriers of the disease. Any horses imported from areas known to suffer from outbreaks of glanders should be tested.

Parasitic manges

There are two types of disease, each caused by a different parasite.

Sarcoptic mange

This disease is caused by the mite Sarcoptes scabei and affects all domestic and farm animals. Man can also be affected, the condition being known as scabies.

Signs

The mites burrow into the skin, causing intense irritation.

The hair drops out in patches.

Lesions form, from which serum exudes.

The skin becomes hardened and folded.

Progressive emaciation may lead to death.

Treatment

A deep skin scrape is taken to confirm the type of mite causing the condition. Saturating parasiticide sprays may then be used as directed by the vet. The vet may also recommend the use of short-wave (gamma) radiation.

Psoroptic mange

There are two types; one affecting the ear, the other affecting the skin. The parasite involved, Psoroptes equi, reproduces rapidly, so stringent control is necessary.

Signs

The mites bite the skin but do not penetrate. However, the irritation leads to the horse rubbing and causing further damage. Bare patches form on the body, often at the base of the mane and tail. The bare patches turn into lesions and exude serum which forms a moist scab in which the parasites live.

Treatment
This is the same as for sarcoptic mange.

Rabies

Rabies is the Latin word for 'madness'. This highly contagious disease occurs in every continent of the world except Australasia and Antarctica. It affects all mammals and, occasionally, birds. It can be transmitted from animal to human, although the horse is usually the end host.

Causes
Rabies is caused by a Lyssavirus which is transmitted in saliva. When it has gained entrance into the body tissue, for example as the result of a bite, the virus travels along the nerve fibres to the central nervous system.

The virus may be present in the saliva before the animal shows any actual signs of the disease. The time taken for signs to show varies from approximately three weeks to three months — this is partially dependent upon the quantity of virus present in the saliva.

Signs
Inflammation around the bite wound — the animal bites and tears at it as a result of intense irritation.

Increased excitement and viciousness, and a general air of derangement, interspersed by periods of calmness.

Also: tremors and muscle spasm, breathing difficulties and hind limb paralysis.

Then recumbency and coma, followed by death.

Rabies is diagnosed upon the clinical signs backed up by laboratory confirmation.

Treatment
A number of vaccines are available to aid prevention but, once contracted, rabies is usually fatal. The horse should be isolated. After death, the brain is examined in the laboratory for confirmation of the diagnosis.

CONCLUSION

A good basic knowledge of equine physiology will assist in choice of horse and adherence to correct training and fitness programmes. These factors will, of themselves, help minimize the likelihood of injury or disease. However, in the event of either occurring, a knowledge of physiology will assist the horse owner or keeper in reporting the matter accurately to the vet, in understanding veterinary diagnosis and prognosis and in following instructions regarding treatment.

Therefore, while such knowledge will maximize the horse owner's chance of having a sound, healthy horse to ride, the ultimate beneficiary will be the most important one... the horse himself.

BIBLIOGRAPHY

Goody, Peter. *Horse Anatomy*. J.A. Allen, 1986.

Johnston, A.M. *Equine Medical Disorders*. Blackwell Scientific Publications, 1986.

Pilliner, Sarah. *Getting Horses Fit*. Collins Professional Books, 1987.

Roberts, M.B.V. *Biology — A Functional Approach*. Thomas Nelson and Sons Ltd., 1979.

Rossdale, P.D. and Wreford, S.M. *The Horse's Health From A to Z*. David and Charles, 1989.

Smythe R.H. and Goody P.C. *The Horse Structure and Movement*. J.A. Allen, 1979.

Snow, Dr. H.H. and Vogel, C.J. *Equine Fitness — The Care and Training of the Athletic Horse*. David and Charles, 1987.

.

INDEX